"OLY 4 KiDS"

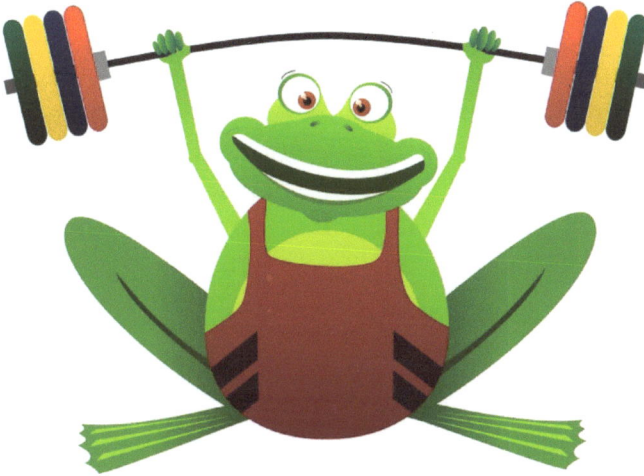

Part 1 - Achieve The Bar

Written by Dani Waller

Characters designed by Karl Moyse
and Zion Waller
Editing by Lauren Moore
Cover re-design by Maddi Wu

Www.Oly4Kids.com.au
For orders, please email: info@oly4kids.com.au

Disclaimer:

The advice and strategies found within may not be suitable for every situation. This work is sold with the understanding that neither the author nor the publisher is held responsible for the results accrued from the advice in this book.

Dedication

I dedicate this book to my three
kids—Jetson, Zion, and Indi.

Everything I do is for you. Xxx

I also dedicate this book to the
great sport of weightlifting and
all the awesome people I have met
through it!

Oly4Kids

Table of Contents

Acknowledgments

I have so many people I could acknowledge here because I have been blessed with having many great people influence my life.

First, I should acknowledge the people who have taught me about weightlifting. Bob Pavone, my first coach, Jack Walls, Javan Waller, Paul Coffa, Michael Keelan, Lyn Jones, Andrew Saxton, Robert Kabbas, Robert Mitchell, Miles Wydall, Angela Wydall, Erin Haff and many, many more.

Secondly, I want to acknowledge the people who believed in me enough to convince me that I should write this book. Roxanne Walker, Ryan Woodall, Suzanne Tilbrook, Narelle Gaunt, Kelliann Brady, Jamie Wilson, and Coral Quinell.

Thirdly, to Karl Moyse and Zion Waller, thanks for all your work on the characters and artwork.

And last but not least, to the kids whom I have already introduced to "Oly 4 Kids". Thanks for your enthusiasm and abilities, which gave me the courage to go forward.

Introduction

When you find your passion in life, you know it! Life will draw you to it, over and over. Weightlifting is my passion in life. That, and my kids—I love my kids. I love all kids in fact. They are so cool and so much fun. Kids are just little people, and they want to try everything the adults do. When something is complicated or overwhelming, it is good practice to break it down into bite-sized chunks. But from another perspective, you need to be very specific and sometimes pedantic to make it safe for all. With those two thoughts in mind, I knew I needed to find a way to "chunk down" and "safe up" the Olympic weightlifting movements so that they are suitable for kids. That's what set me on the path of creating the Oly 4 Kids programme.

When I say "weightlifting", I mean Olympic Weightlifting. There are many different interpretations of the word "weightlifting". But I mean the word in its purest form—the weightlifting that has been performed at the Olympics since its beginnings. Weightlifting was included in the first Olympics in 1896, but as a field event. It only became its own event in 1920. In 1972 the weightlifting competition became what it is today: the snatch and clean & jerk. But it wasn't until the Sydney Olympics in the very recent year of 2000 that the sport included women's categories, at this level.

The year 2000 was a pivotal year for weightlifting, as a trainer named Greg Glassman created a new fitness program called CrossFit. CrossFit has taken the world by storm and brought many people into the gym (or "box" as they are called). CrossFit combines numerous activities into a WOD (workout of the day), one of them being weightlifting. Anyone who has tried a WOD will tell you the Oly movements are very taxing, especially if they are not done with optimal technique. ("Oly' is short for Olympic weightlifting. Many die hard weightlifting fans don't like the term, but it is very contemporary, so I use it.) In fact, it didn't take people long to come to the conclusion that learning Olympic weightlifting techniques would help them in getting ahead in CrossFit. Then another thing happened. These sporty and competitive people found Oly lifting addictive!—just like it has always been for me.

So, kids in weightlifting – a contentious issue? Plenty of parents are concerned that lifting is dangerous and might stunt their child's growth. Are these arguments valid? I've researched and practiced Olympic weightlifting for years now and have come to the conclusion that if you have the proper knowledge and training, Oly lifting is not only safe for kids, but it will help them grow stronger as well. I'm hoping that after reading this book, you too will see the benefits it can have for children.

The most important key to making weightlifting not only safe, but also beneficial in so many ways, is learning the correct technique. And for children, technique is even more essential. The programme I have designed intends to do just that—but with a lot of fun! Kids have a short attention span, so information should be taught in small bursts, intermingled with games and exercise. The programme is broken up into different parts, part 1 being "Achieve the Bar". It takes 10 weeks (of one 45-minute session per week) to complete the whole of part 1. This book covers just Part 1.

I have written this book with the assumption that the reader will already have an understanding and an appreciation for the two weightlifting moves that we are teaching in Oly 4 Kids, being the snatch and the clean & jerk. If you don't have this knowledge, you may want to get a quick crash course or at least an overview to be able to understand what we are teaching here.

The programme is intended for Primary School age kiddos, although I have had students as young as two years old—and doing well, I might add!

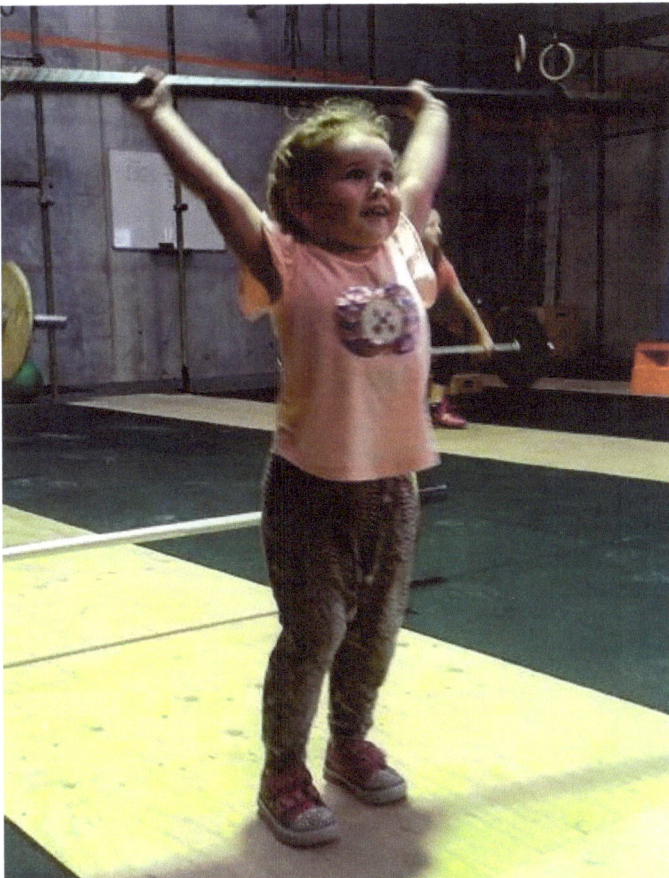

Equipment

To start the programme, you don't need anything. But pretty soon you will need either broomsticks, wooden poles, or narrow plastic pipes for your child to practice on. The pole just needs to be light and narrow enough that a child can fit his or her hands around it. Blocks of some sort would be handy, so your child can set the bar down at the same height it would be at if it had rubber bumper weights on each end. Better still, round plywood discs the size and height of rubber bumper plates, able to be fitted on the poles, are great! If you know anyone handy enough to make these, be sure to get two for each bar.

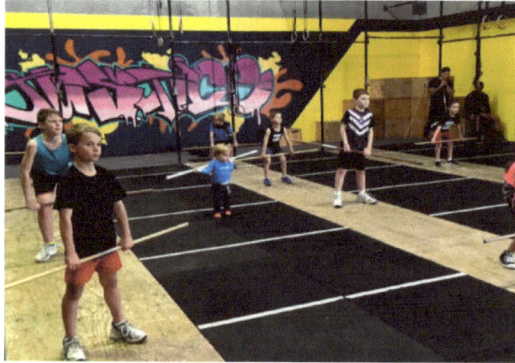

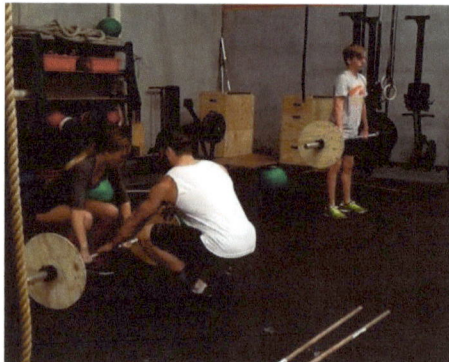

In Part 2, you will need to acquire 8kg technique bars that look like weightlifting bars but are made of a lighter material. Also, low squat racks would be handy, but you can use teaching assistants or parents to stand there as weight racks.

Eventually, it would be ideal to have the larger sized light weight plastic bumper plates that come in 2.5 kg and 5 kg. However, they won't be needed until Part 2 or even Part 3.

Attire

Obviously, parents may want to avoid spending any money upfront, if possible. But there are certain items that will help your child succeed.

Olympic weighting shoes have a raised, hard heel on them to assist the athlete to be in the right position, and to be stable and able to impart force with the movements.

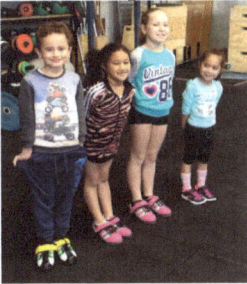

Proper shoes can be expensive and hard to find. Clothes should be fitted and comfortable. The squat positions are not dainty, so wearing either bike shorts or booty shorts would be best, or longer shorts for boys. Weightlifters wear a one-piece suit in competition, but we can leave that until later. ☺

Safety

When an excited bunch of kids gets together, expect an abundance of energy and light-hearted mayhem. Put a few wooden poles into the mix and this could spell disaster! So right up front, at the beginning of every session, I always lay down a few ground rules. First and foremost, whenever the kids are moving around with a practice bar, they must walk and hold the pole in the middle, vertically. It is not a lightsabre, a sword, or a spear. And they will think of this. Even a few adults I know have taught the basics to have come up with this idea. (Let's face it—adults are just big kids a lot of the time!)

Secondly, in every exercise we do, each child must have plenty of space around them in case they get unbalanced (again: the wooden pole) or even just body crash. Let's save the energy for the Oly!

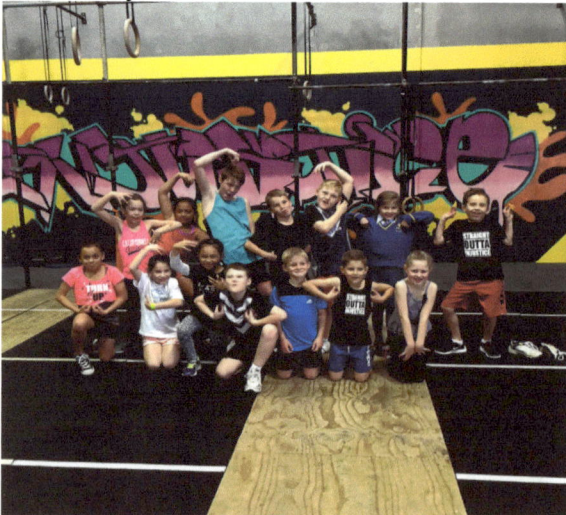

Part 1 - Achieve the Bar

Overview

The key to good technique is to learn the proper positions and the movements without any weight involved. This principle is true for adults and kids, although it is very hard to convince some adults of this point, especially the male variety! But with kids, it is imperative. So Part 1 is all about that—learning the positions and the movements. The challenge here is to keep the child's attention and to make it fun, while still ensuring that the kids get the movements right. For this reason, I have come up with fun names for each of the learned disciplines, mostly by using animals. Kids love pretending to be animals, and with the help of a few crazy characters and this book, I will teach you and your child each of the correct Oly positions and movements.

This book also includes progress cards and charts for the lifting coaches to use. Kids love visual evidence of their progress and success. When a child completes a level, I take a photo of the student holding a placard saying, "I passed …" Not only do the kids love this acknowledgement, but the parents do too. To pass each level, I have compiled a checklist that must be completed. You can find the checklist at the end of each section.

Some children will learn the moves very quickly, even immediately. So to be able to give students the chance to master each move, intermingle instruction with games. I have suggestions for such games, but you can make up some yourself as well. The objective is to make the student repeat the movement over and over, without it seeming monotonous.

It is also advantageous to make it necessary to hold certain positions to build muscle strength and flexibility, as well as muscle memory.

Music is really important! It creates a fun atmosphere and gives a cadence to the movements and positions. And it just makes you feel good. Incorporating music and movement has always been a fantastic strategy for keeping you motivated while you learn and develop.

We also want to keep the mind healthy. By that I mean to always give out positive reinforcement. If you need to criticize something, first comment on a good point. You know what they say—for every one piece of negative feedback, a child needs about ten times the amount of positive feedback. In education they call this "sandwiching". You "sandwich" a negative or corrective comment in between positives. So reiterate the positive point to finish with what went well. And try to correct only one thing at a time until they get comfortable with that. It is hard, I know, if you see numerous movement errors at once. But you will lose them if you just rattle off four or five things for them to fix. Correct one thing and see how they cope with that before you decide to point out another thing for them to think about. All kids are different, of course. The smarter or older kids may be quicker at picking things up, so you can give them more instruction than you would to another child. But this programme allows all the kids to move at their own pace, as games and refreshers along the way give everyone extra time to practise, if needed.

Above all, make it fun. Allow the kids to laugh and goof around—and goof around with them! This will only increase their level of progress. So, let's get into the programme!

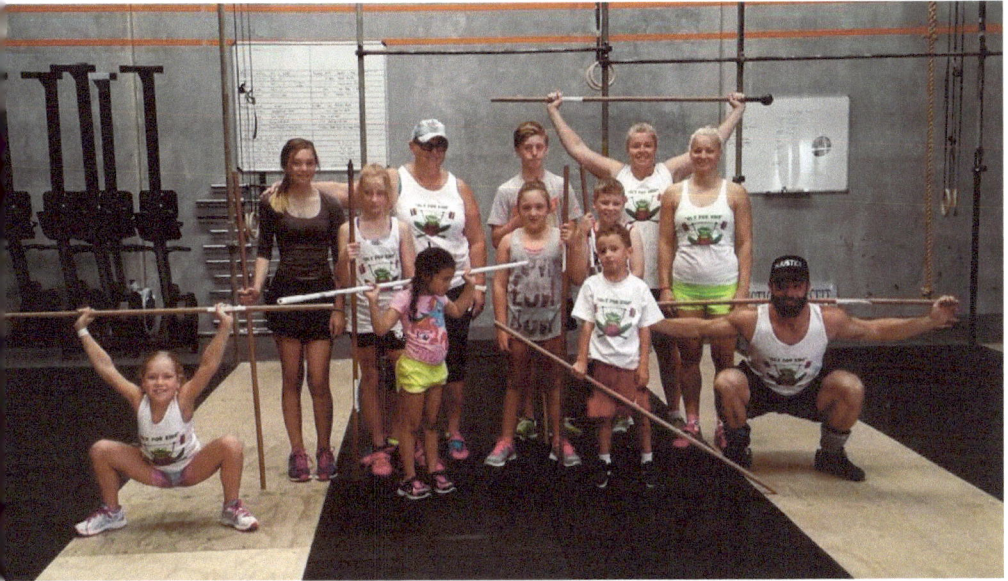

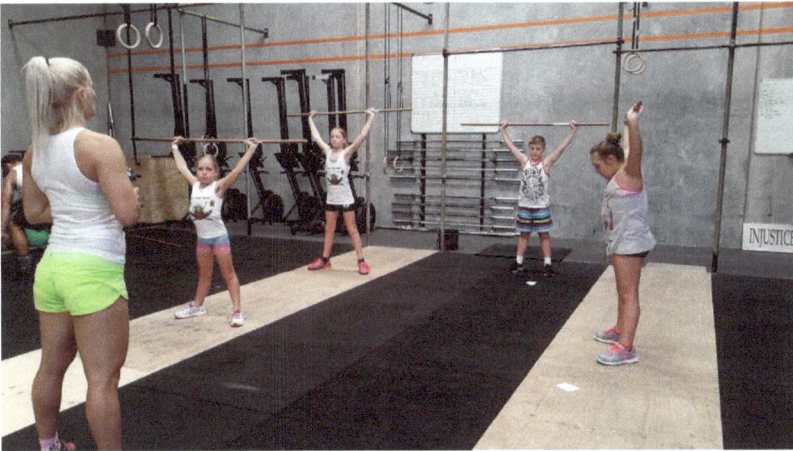

Oly4Kids

1. The Standing Monkey

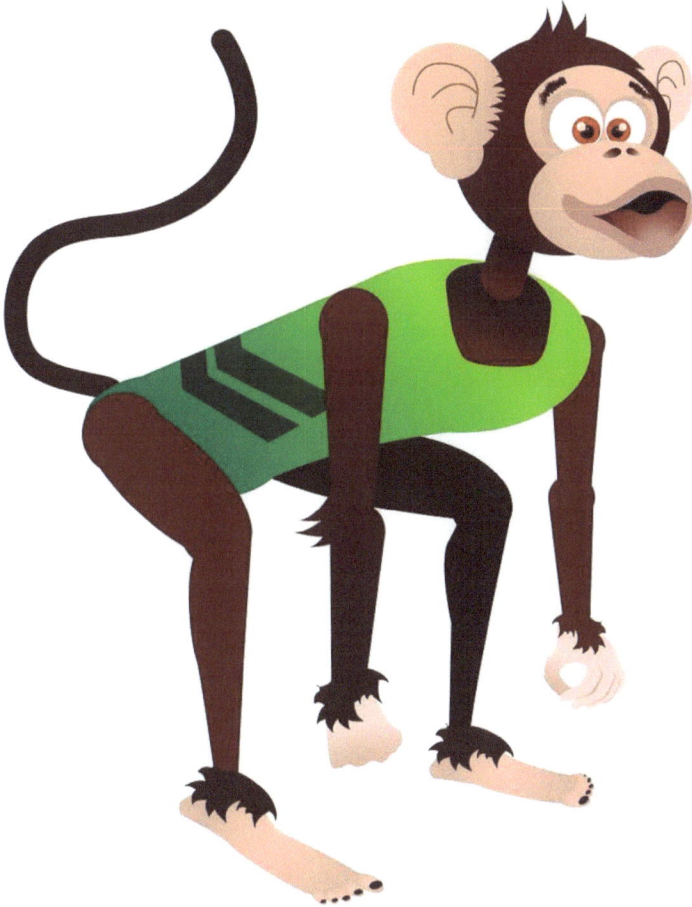

Ha! The Standing Monkey—that just sounds funny, doesn't it? Well, it is important to make this bit funny and really spend some time on it. The standing monkey is the starting position, relevant to both the snatch and the clean & jerk. It is the foundation for both lifts, and if you don't get this right to start with, you will find everything else very difficult, to say the least.

The standing monkey is all about strength, core stability, and centering.

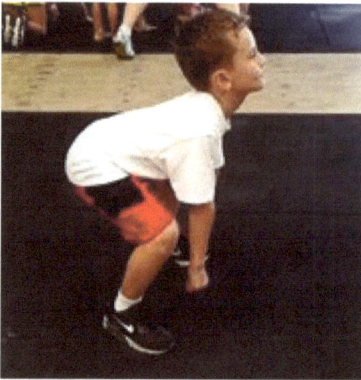

Finding the right start position is imperative in order to move the bar off the ground and in a straight, efficient line. Many sports scientists have spent a great deal of time studying this movement, and there is a lot of literature on it if you want to learn more about it. But to keep it simple, the back must be flat and at about a 45-degree angle. The thighs should be a 45-degree angle downward. I have always felt like a monkey or a gorilla when I hold this position, so that is how I teach it to kids. It makes them laugh, and you can have a lot of fun playing around with it. The chest must be forward and over the bar while keeping the shoulders back. Knees and feet should be turned outward.

That is a lot of information to give a kid all at once, so if you need to chunk it down, do so. Teach them to keep their backs flat, and walk around like a monkey. Play a game, and once they seem to be getting that posture, instruct them to keep their knees out. And so on.

Once all of these bits of information are passed on to the kids, teach them about the **hook grip**. This grip is fundamental to lifting weights effectively and safely, so teach it now, at the beginning. And remember—students can learn all of these positions without a bar or pole of any sort.

Hook grip is where you first wrap the thumb around the bar, and then the rest of the fingers around the bar, <u>over the top</u> of the thumb. The reason for this is because it enhances the grip you have on the bar, as the fingers over the top hold the thumb in place and the bar at the same time. It has the same effect as putting a wrap around the bar to help with grip. This won't seem important now as we are not going to be pulling any significant weight for some time in this programme. But it is really important to form good habits from the beginning. This is one position I have found really difficult in convincing adults who are new to the sport to do.

Here are a few games to play with the kids to get them to practice the monkey stand and help them feel comfortable in this starting position.

Musical Monkeys

This game is much like musical chairs, except there are no chairs. When the music stops, everyone must drop to the standing monkey position and hold it. Take your time choosing who was the last person to drop, because this gives them a chance to hold the position, and you can make corrections of the position where needed. Whoever was last to drop into position is out and has to sit down. And of course, the last monkey standing is the winner. I suggest you have lots of practice rounds before you start eliminating, as this makes sure that everyone gets in lots of practice.

This game is always a favourite and can be played week after week as a fun warm-up.

Pick up the Bananas

This game can be played with or without equipment, but you need stations where the "bananas" are to be picked up. If you want to use equipment, set up wooden poles on blocks at the height that a weightlifting bar would be at if it had rubber bumpers attached. You want to play this game at two different bar grips: narrow (the clean grip) and wide (the snatch grip). So half of the banana stations will have blocks spaced out widely so the bar can be picked up with a narrow (clean) grip. The other half of the blocks should be placed closer together so the bar can be picked up with a wide (snatch) grip.

There are a number of ways to play this game: one way is to have four banana stations at one end of the gym, and four lines of kids at the other. When the music starts the first person runs to the bar (banana station), stand in front of the bar, and picks up the bar with a hook grip. One of the coaches will say it's good and the bar is put back on the blocks and the kid will run over to the next line. You keep it going until all kids have picked up all bars. With music, the kids find this activity to be a lot of fun. No winners are needed, but if you need to make it a competition, find out who has the best monkey stand.

Monkey Stare Down

This game is played in pairs. Have the children face each other in the standing monkey position. The coach calls out instructions like "right hand on your head" or "monkey stand". Mix it up with stuff like "act like a monkey" or "call out your name". If you don't hold the position that was last called until the next call, you are out. It is a lot of fun because the kids are facing each other. Every now and then you can get them to run to the wall and back to stop fatigue.

Finally, when you feel most of the class knows this position, you can test them with the following list:

Checklist to Pass "The Standing Monkey"

- Feet apart
- Knees turned outward
- Hook grip
- Flat back (stick bottom out)
- Chest over bar
- Looking forward.

If you laminate this checklist and put it on a clipboard, you can tick it off as they show you the moves.

When all items are ticked, let them celebrate and take a photo of them holding the
"I have passed the Standing Monkey" sign.

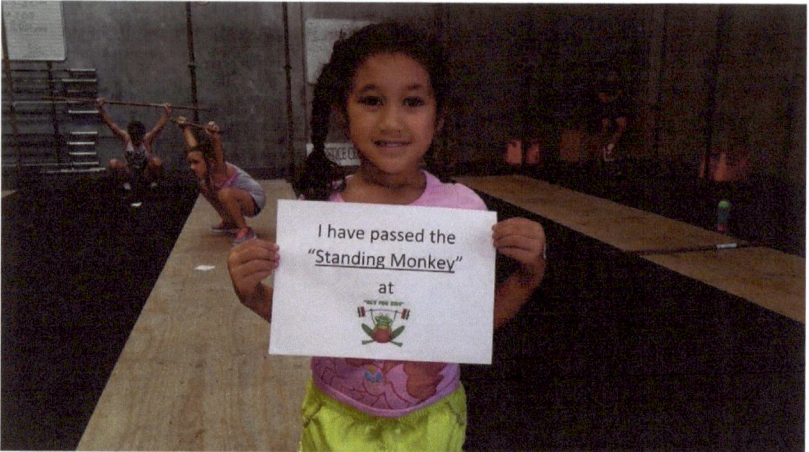

2. *Stretchy Cat*

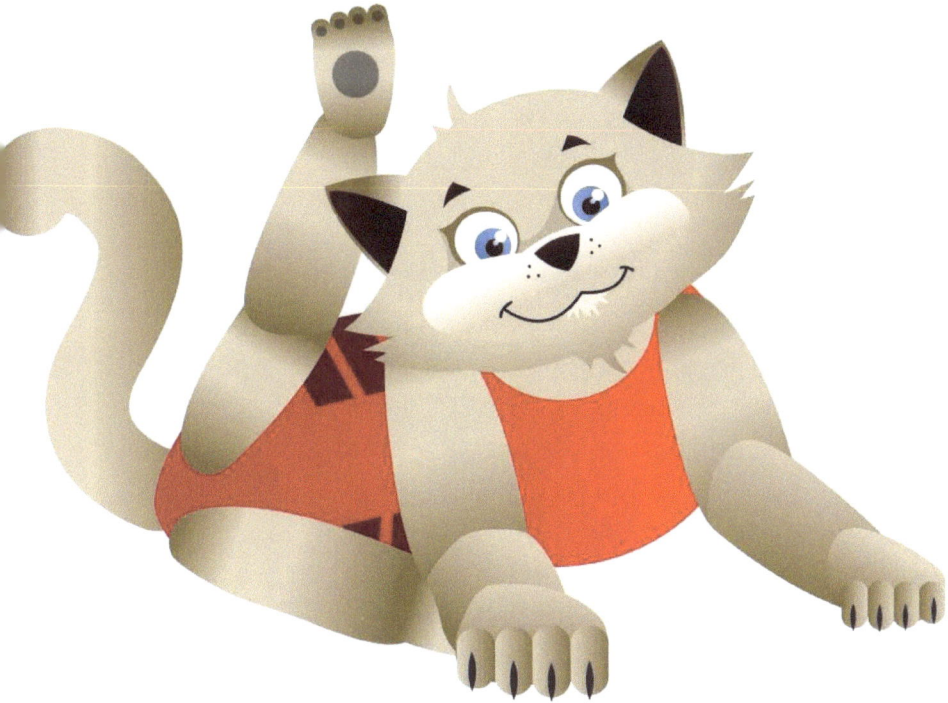

Stretchy Cat is actually the last level to pass on ***Achieve the Bar***, but it is important to practice these movements at the end of every class for 5 to 10 minutes, so we are going to cover it now.

This level entails stretching out all the muscles that we contract and tighten while lifting so that we can alleviate soreness and tightness later. Kids are way more supple than adults, but it is still important for them to go through these movements at the end of every class, for a number of reasons. Firstly, it will stretch out the muscles used. Secondly, it can be a bit of fun

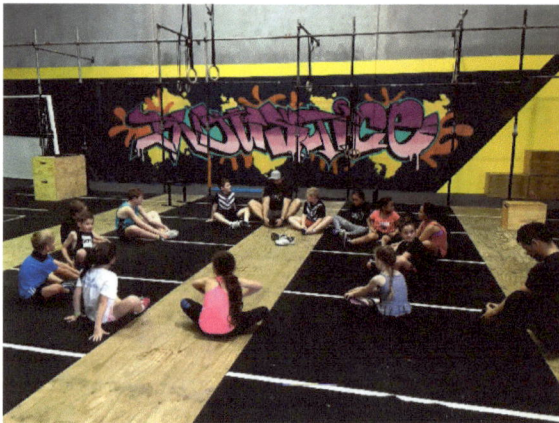

to sit together in a circle, connect with the kids, and have a laugh. Point out the kids who can do certain stretches well; quite often they are the same kiddos who may have struggled with other parts of Oly. It is a nice way to finish the class, on a happy note. Thirdly, and the most important reason to me, learning to stretch now instils good habits in the kids that will stay with them as they grow older. Stretching is one aspect of exercise that is neglected because it doesn't seem as important on the surface. But stretching really is key to muscle growth and balance—especially for the boys. They are the ones that will gain the most from it. So teach good habits from the get-go.

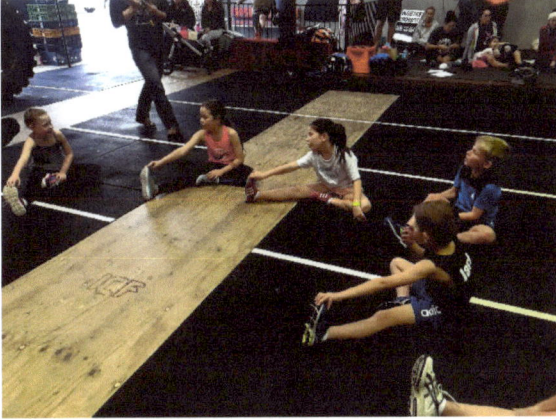

I haven't got a Sports Science degree so I am going to keep this nice and simple using layman's terms. My apologies to those of you who have the professional expertise to discuss this area better, but I am just going to give my readers a general overview. Mobility and flexibility are such important topics and could probably have a book of their own.

Here are some suggestions for some stretches you can do.

The Praying Mantis: Squat down with your elbows pushing out on your knees and your hands in a praying position. This stretches the inner thigh area, the lower back, and the upper back. It is important to keep the back flat, chest high, and your butt sticking out (not curled under).

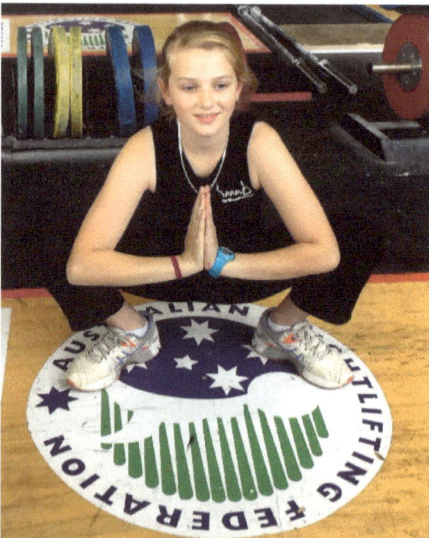

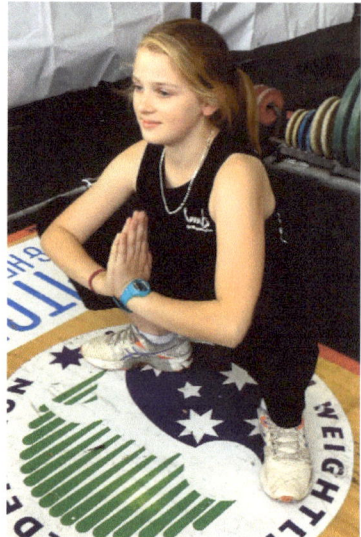

The Straddle: Sit on the ground with your legs outward, as

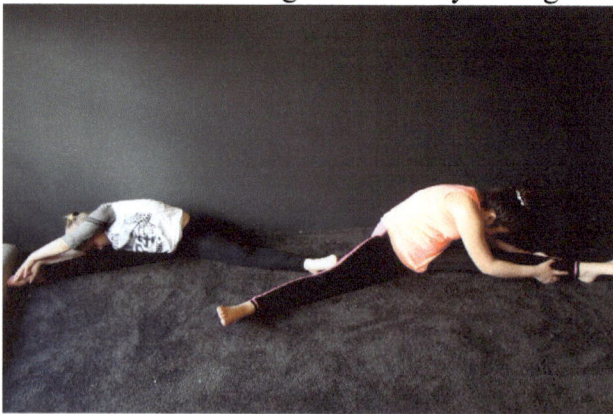

far apart as you can get them. For the more flexible kids, get them to push their chest towards the ground. Then show them how to stretch down each leg, reaching towards to the foot.

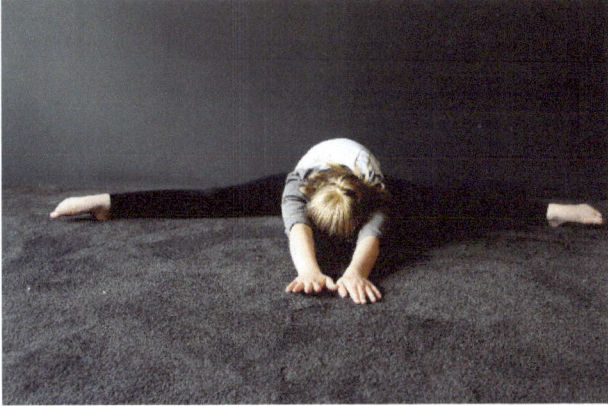

The Hurdle Stretch: Sit on the ground with one leg forward and the other bent at the knee to the side and behind you. Then

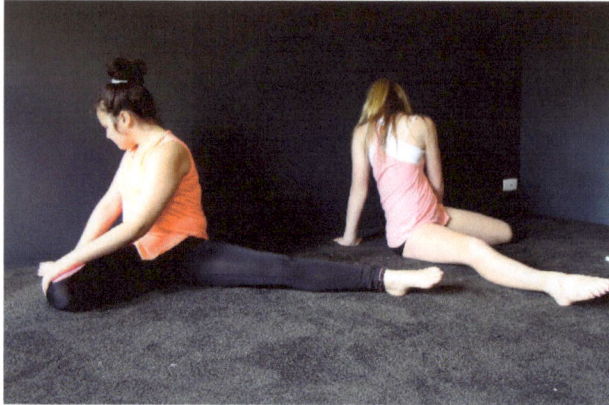

stretch around across your straight leg first as far as you can. I tell the kids to look at their bottom. That gets them to stretch as far as they can. Then you twist back across your bent leg as far as you can. Same again, ask the kids to look at their bottom. This stretches the back as well as the quads.

The Superman Stretch: This one is a beauty but must be done under strict supervision. Get the kids to pair up with someone of a similar size. Then one person lies on the ground face down with their arms extended forward and out (like a "V"). The second person picks up the first person's arms and slowly and carefully pulls them up and back. Like Superman flying (hence the name). This stretch is held for about 10 seconds and then carefully placed back down. When I do this stretch with adults, I get them to do it in a jerk position and then a snatch position, but because the kids haven't learnt this yet, we just do one position.

This stretch can also be done standing between a doorway or holding onto two poles (at the correct width). Also, kids can do this with their parents at home where the parents hold the arms and the child either steps or leans forward.

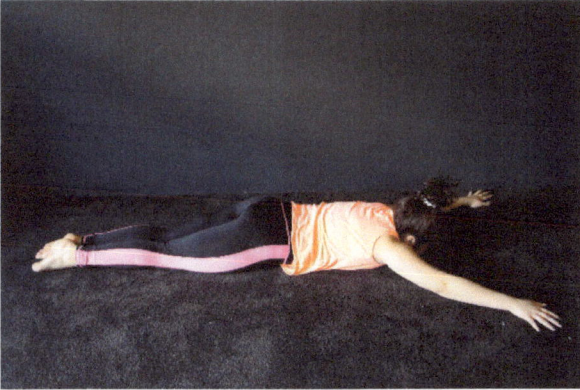

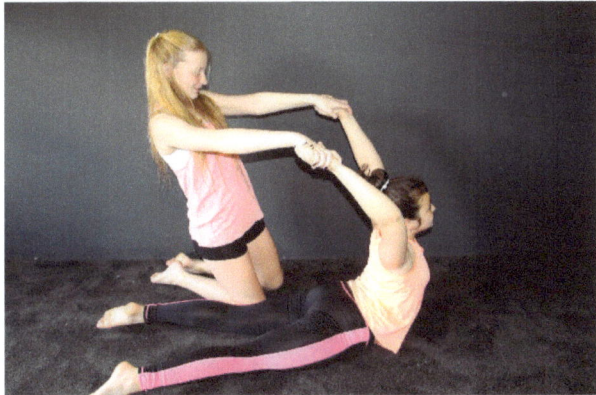

The purpose of this stretch is to open up the shoulders and increase the mobility in the shoulder region. It is vital for the moves coming up, in order for the lifters to be able to gain maximum advantage.

The Box Stretch: Put one leg up on a box, bend that knee (like a lunge), and then lean forward to stretch the inner thigh. Change legs and do the same on the other side.

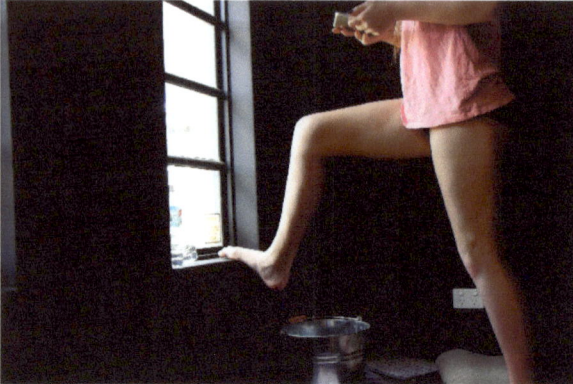

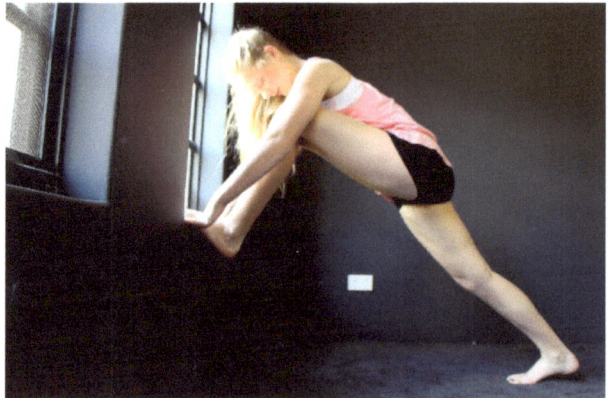

The Back Twist: I am sure there is a more technical term for this one, but this is what I call it. Lie on your back with your arms stretched outward. Raise one leg and point your toe to the opposite knee. Then push that bent knee over the straight leg as far as you can, as close to the ground on the other side. You must keep both shoulders on the ground while you are doing this twist. Hold it for 10 seconds or so to get a good stretch in your back happening. You can use the opposite arm

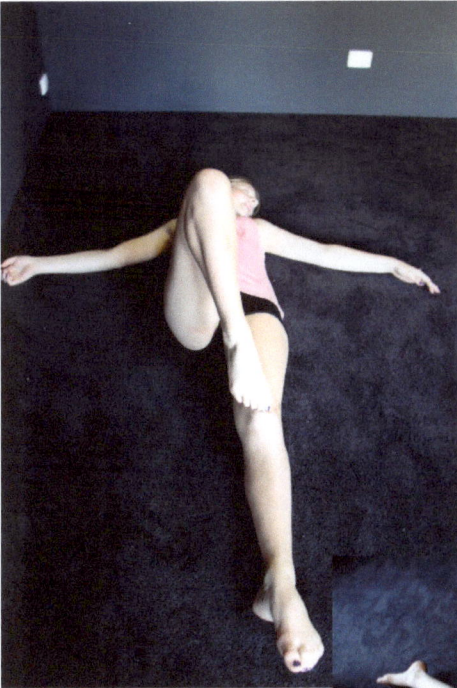

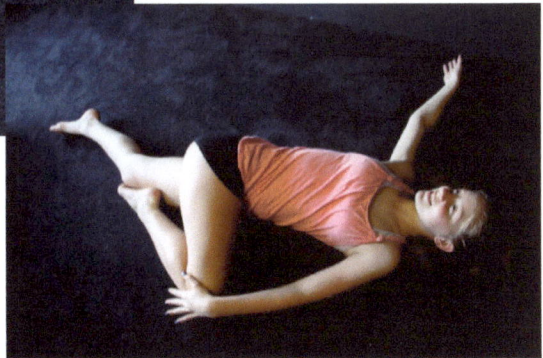

to the knee to help pull it over to maximize the stretch. Then do the same on the other side, with the opposite leg and hand.

The Squashed Frog: This is another stretch that must be properly supervised! Get the kids to lay on their front with their legs out to the sides and bent, so the toes come back together. This stretches the inner thighs and is a killer. But kids are much more supple than adults and may be able to do this easily. But you must make sure there is no stray kids mucking around that think it would be a good idea to jump on someone's back while doing a "squashed frog"—that could be bad!

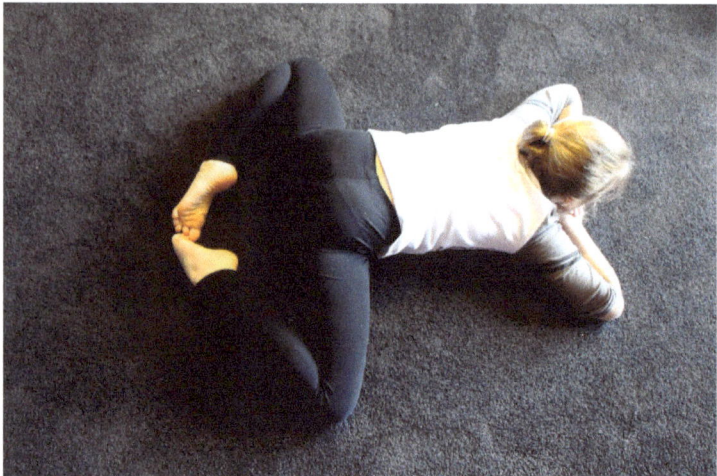

3. The Proud Grasshopper

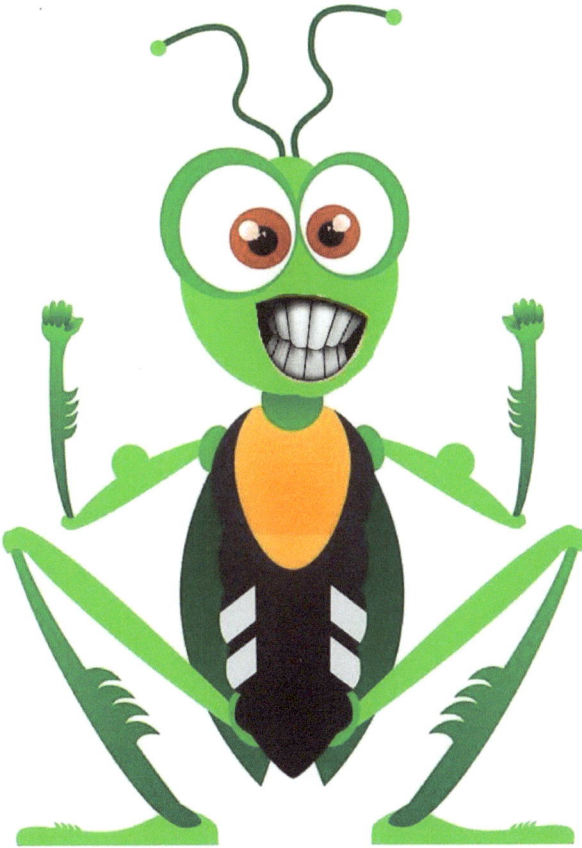

The next move that needs to be taught is the front squat position. That name doesn't sound like a lot of fun. So we call it the "Proud Grasshopper". There is so much about this position that reminds me of a grasshopper. Firstly, the legs have to be bent so far that they practically double over. The knees need to stay over the feet and out, to allow the hips to come in as close to your heels as possible. This keeps the lifter centered and balanced. But the position does require a lot of flexibility. Now with kids, this is not such a problem. You can usually teach this position pretty easily to most children

.

The "proud" part of the name reminds the child to keep the chest big and the chin up, parallel to the ground. This must all be done without allowing the child to round the back. This can cause injury and long-term damage if it is allowed.

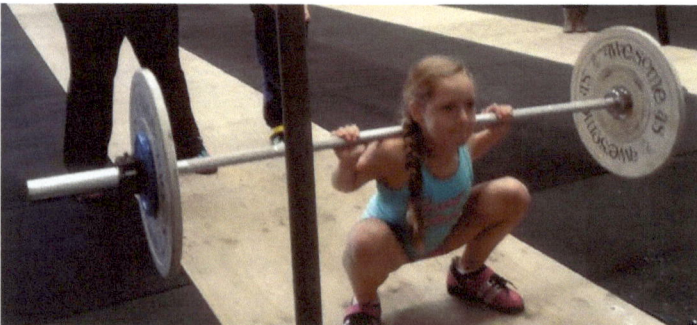

So, the back must be flat with the bottom sticking out, not

tucked under (we call this "butt wink"). The chest must be out, shoulders back. First teach the position with a wooden pole across the back of the neck, in the back squat position. And to maintain a good squat position, make sure the lifter has her knees out and forward over the feet.

Then teach that position the same but with the bar in front of the lifter's neck. When the bar is in front of the neck, the elbows must be high and pointed forward. This will be covered more in the Torpedo Elbows section.

There are three key aspects of the Proud Grasshopper position that must be taught, one at a time.
Firstly, this position must be learnt static and held. Assist the child into the position and talk her through all the points that are important. She can hold that position while you are correcting it to get it right, so she can learn muscle memory and mobility.

Next, the lifter needs to be taught to drop into it fast. The position should be planned right from the standing position so as the child drops fast into the position with her back straight, bottom pushing out, and chest kept high.

Lastly, you will want the kids to try to bounce out of this position at the bottom—to just dip down into it and jump straight back up. This is the starting position for squats—front squats, to be exact. And it is also the start of doing a clean. This requires them learning to "catch the bounce" at the bottom of the squat. While this movement is pretty hard for older athletes to master, it is relatively easy for children to learn. Hence, we teach this movement early.

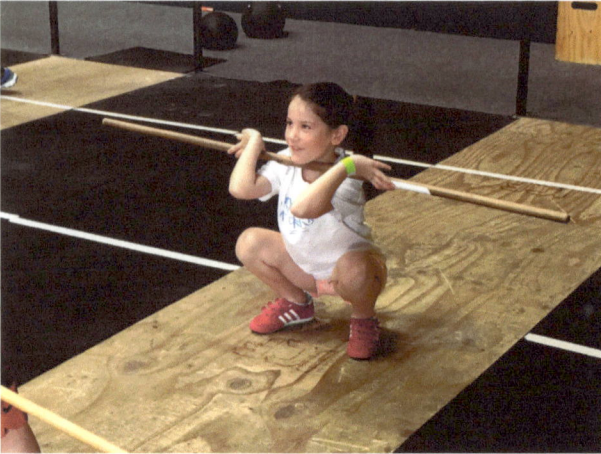

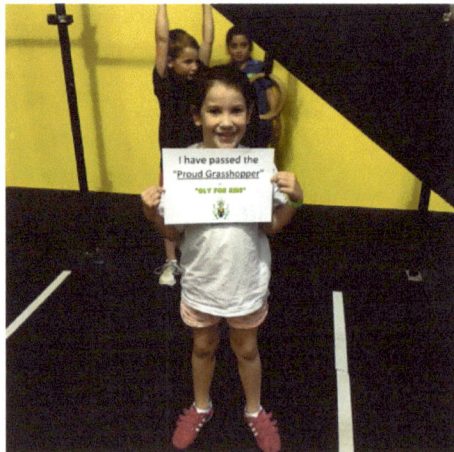

Here are a few games to play with the kids to practice the Proud Grasshopper and to get them to feel comfortable in this squat position.

Musical Monkeys and Grasshoppers

This game is just an extended version of Musical Monkeys, with the addition of Proud Grasshoppers. So when the music stops, you can either call out one of the two positions randomly, or you can have a coaching assistant do one of the moves and have everyone copy it. You could even add in that the child with the best position in one round can choose the character in the next round. I think you get the drift: get the kids to repeat the moves and hold them, over and over again.

Proud Grasshopper Ladder

For this activity, set up a course or ladder of exercise stations. You need five places: the first one is for the back squat, the second is the front squat, the third is the jump front squat (fast drop), the fourth and the fifth are for catching the bounce. If you make the fifth station close to the fourth, they can actually jump straight from the fourth to the fifth, if they are good! This activity design creates a challenge of balance and core stability. If you get the kids to cycle through this course about five times, they will lock into the technique and feel of the Proud Grasshopper right away.

Finally, when you feel most of the class knows this position, you can test them with the following list:

Checklist to Pass "The Proud Grasshopper"

- Feet apart
- Knees outward
- Hands on shoulders
- Bottom close to ankles
- BIG Chest
- Looking forward.

4. The Jumping Frog

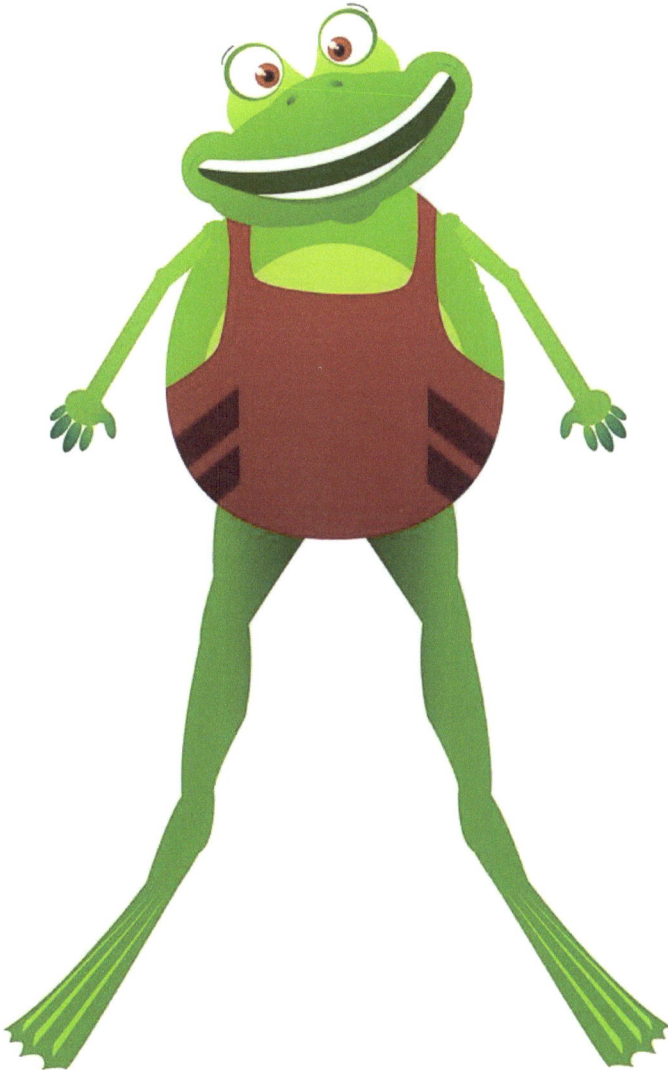

The Jumping Frog is a really important component of both Oly lifts, in that it is important to grasp the concept that you are jumping, with straight arms, not *putting* the bar on your chest or overhead. To get the most out of both the snatch and the clean & jerk, the initial pulling the bar off the ground is where all the momentum and speed comes from. So rather than thinking you are pulling the bar off the ground to place it, know that you are exploding off the ground to then catch the bar in its receiving position. If you can get this idea into your head before you start the full lifts, you will have a much better start. So let the kids learn to jump. And jump like a frog, because they have to come from a semi-squatting position (the standing monkey), so it feels a lot like you are a frog. And if you get it right, you will look like a frog in mid-flight.

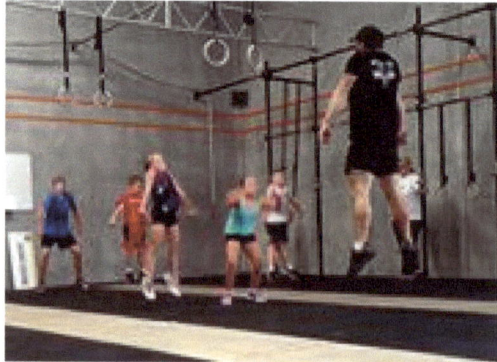

The first thing I tell the kids is to imagine a frog. A frog has a big chest and the chest lifts first and leads the way. You would never see a frog lift its bottom in the air! So if someone does that (adults do it all the time!), ask the kids if they've ever seen a frog lift their bottom to jump. No, they haven't – frogs always use their legs to push upwards and off the ground.

But there are a few preparatory things you need to teach students before they can jump like a frog. First, instruct them to lock their elbows. When they first go to lift something, most people automatically bend their elbows to use the arm muscles to lift it. But the arm muscles are not as strong as the leg, core, and back muscles. So when pulling the bar, or lifting it off the ground, you want to use those stronger muscles instead. And the best way to do that is to disengage the arm muscles by locking them in line. If you lock the elbows straight, then the arms act as a pendulum rather than a moving part. If you turn the outside of the elbow up and lock it tight, then when you pull the bar, it won't bend. Try it yourself.

Here are a few games to play with the kids to help them practice the Jumping Frog and get the feel of the jump.

Highest Jump

Have the kids to line up along the wall and one by one get them to do the biggest jump they can. You can measure on the wall or with objects lined up, how far they can jump and get their feet off the ground. Make a chart or some kind of reference for each child. Next week when you play the same game again, have them compete with their own previous best height. The best measure is against themselves. Don't make some kids feel bad that they are not as athletic as others. Make them feel good about their own improvement.

Musical Monkeys and Frogs

Here's another extended version of Musical Monkeys, although when the music comes back on, ask the kids to make the biggest jump they can from the stationary standing monkey position.

It's good to reinforce skills that we have taught in previous weeks, so any of the games played on previous weeks can be brought back out again. You want to refresh the kiddos' memories and retest skills continually. It also gives the kids a measure and makes them feel good to demonstrate the skills they already know after spending thirty minutes trying to master something new. So, play games they know how to play. Enjoy the fun they've had before. Therefore, your aim is to slowly decrease the time spent learning new skills each week while refreshing known skills more and more often. This brings all the skills together—and that is the whole idea of this part of the programme. First, chunk down all the movements and learn the individual skills… and then put it all together to make the whole Oly movements work efficiently and effectively.

When you feel most of the class knows this skill, you can test them with the following list:

Checklist to Pass the "Jumping Frog"

- Locked elbows
- Keep chest over bar
- Straighten knees
- Squeeze bottom
- Have a tight tummy
- Shrug shoulders

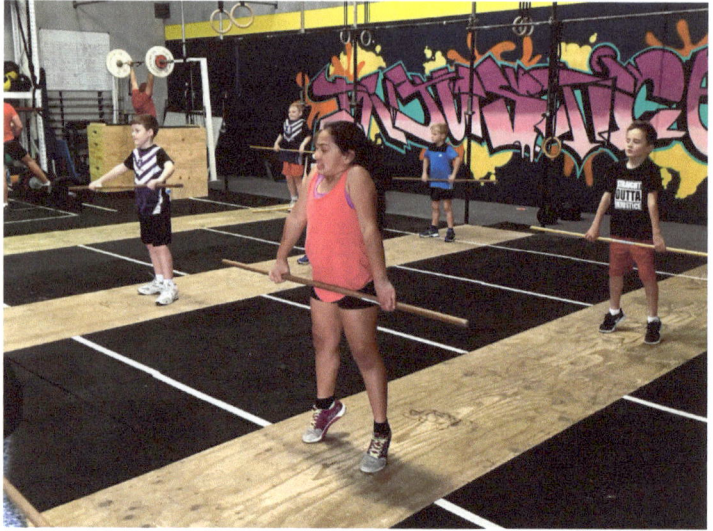

5. *Torpedo Elbows*

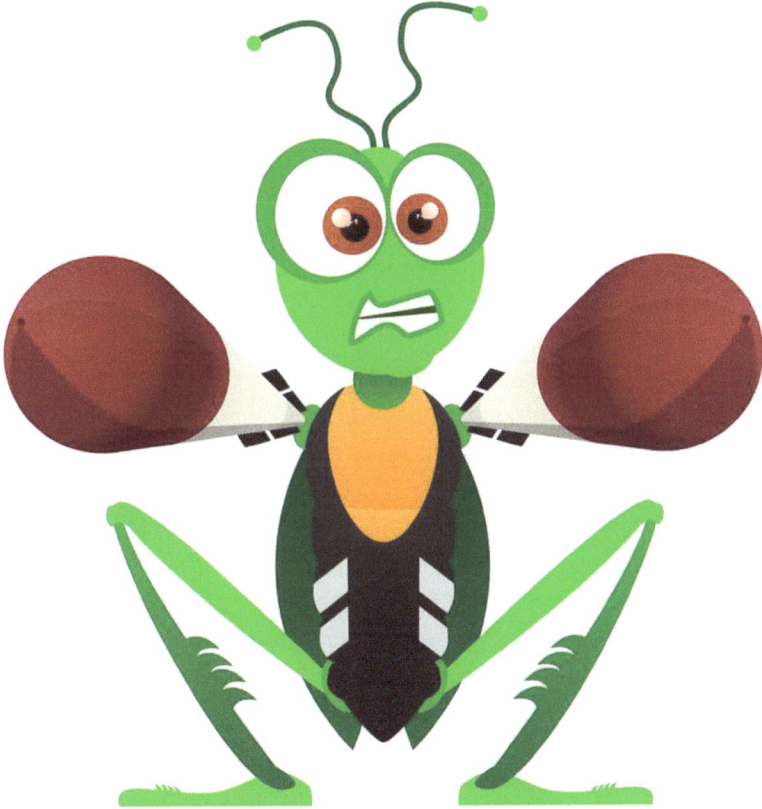

An important part of the clean movement is to keep the elbows high when you're in the full squat position. By this, I mean that your upper arms should be parallel to the ground with your elbows pointing forward much like they would be if you were shooting a torpedo. And that's why we call this position Torpedo Elbows. It's hard to teach a child the correct high arm position. But if you help them to imagine that they can shoot something in front of them with these imaginary torpedoes, then that will help their bodies get into the correct position through the mind-body connection.

To clean correctly, the lifter must get into the position as quickly as possible. The speed at which you achieve "torpedo elbows" is important to the effect. Having high elbows in the full squat position does a few things. It helps to keep (or push) the chest up high, which in turn keeps the back flat. It also makes the bar more stable and easier to hold. What you are trying to achieve is to create a "rack" for the bar to sit on. The bar is held up by your torso, chest, and shoulders, which is why it is called a "rack" position. It is not intended that the bar is held by your hands and arms. They are merely used to direct the bar to the rack position.

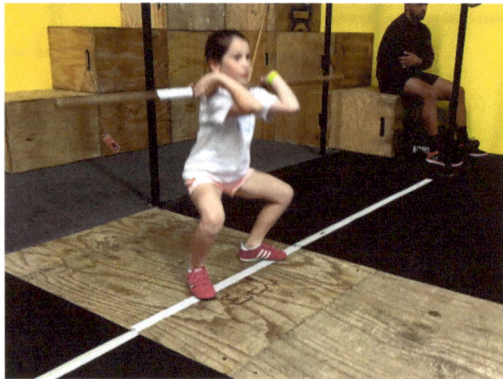

Here are a few games to play with the kids to help them practice the Torpedo Elbows and get the feel of the rack position.

Shoot-Out!

Have the kids stand evenly spread out with their eyes shut. Then ask them to slowly turn around a few times. When you say "stop", they must open their eyes and point "torpedo elbows" at the first person they see. After doing this a few times, you make it a competition, so the slowest torpedo elbows kiddo has to sit down. The rest of the group moves around (with music is probably best), and then you play the game again. And then on the third or fourth round, you eliminate one more person. This will eventually leave you with the fastest draw in the gym. You can mix it up by calling "low draw" and "high draw" so that the "torpedo elbows" are pulled in either the squat position or the standing position, respectively.

Musical Monkeys and Grasshoppers

Here's another extended version of Musical Monkeys. The only difference is that when the music comes back on, ask the kids to make either a standing monkey position or a torpedo elbows grasshopper. You can do this a number of ways. Either call the position ("Monkey!" or "Grasshopper!") when the music stops or have a picture of a standing monkey on one wall and a picture of a proud grasshopper with torpedo elbows on another wall. And whichever wall they see first when the music stops is the position they must drop to. And always make them hold that position for 5 to 10 seconds so they work those muscles.

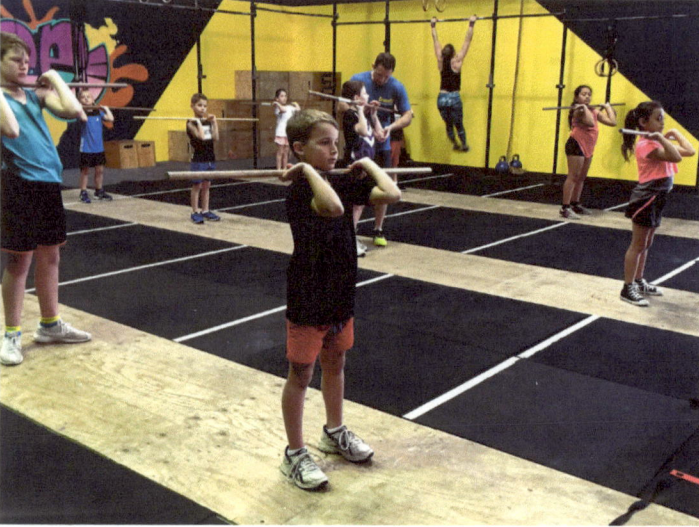

Finally, when you see that the majority of the class knows this skill, you can test them with the following list:

Checklist to Pass "Torpedo Elbows"

- Hands outside shoulders

- Arms parallel to ground

- Chest high

- Squat position

- Stand position

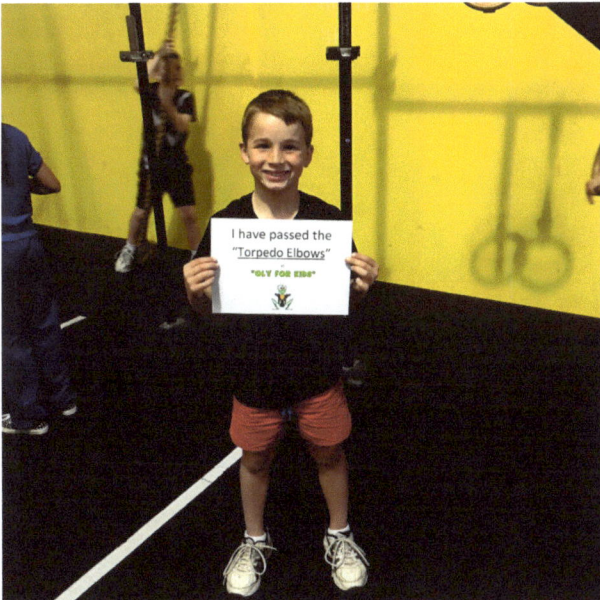

6. *Duck Walks*

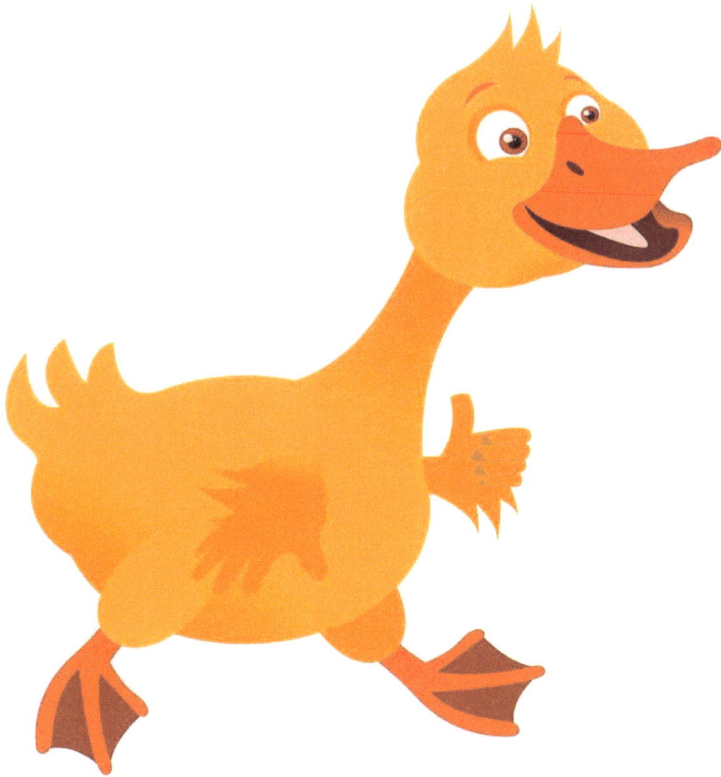

This part of the programme is not something we do in a snatch or a clean & jerk but is more about developing stability in the squat positions. Teach it first by having the children put their hands on their hips so their whole focus is on the feet, hips, and chest. Conduct duck walk relays to give them plenty of time to just be in that position and to learn the feel of having the hips close to the heels. The kids find this one a lot of fun. Let them make quacking noises and act like ducks. We want this to be fun! There is nothing serious about this exercise except for the five learning outcome points, which are:

- Bottom close to your heels
- Keep chest high
- Hands on hips
- Torpedo elbows
- Arms over head

The third, fourth, and fifth point all relate to the three different squat styles. "Hands on hips" is basically just the duck walk position. This position is closest to the back squat form. Changing your hand position from the hips to making torpedo elbows puts you in the front squat position. Then putting your arms overhead is the snatch squat position.

So, duck walks—why? We're not going to walk like a duck when lifting, so why would we do it now? It is because we are teaching lifters the positions, mobility, core stability, and balance necessary to doing the Oly lifts later. Practicing the duck walk will accomplish that. And—which is just as important—the kids are having fun.

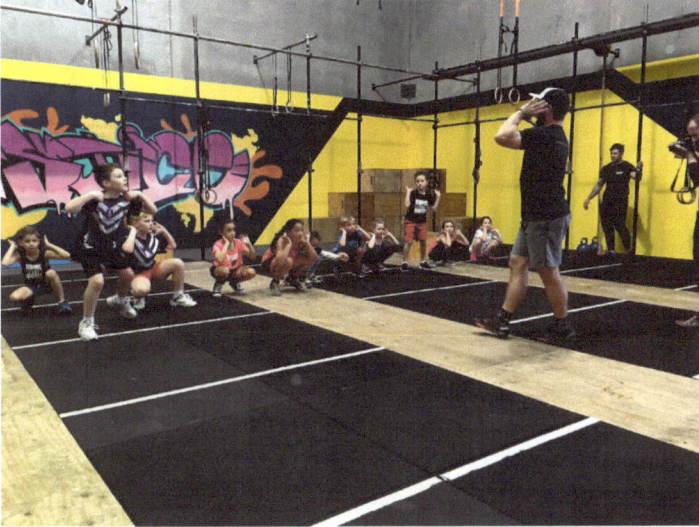

Here are a few games to play with the kids to help them practice the Duck Walks and get the feel of that deep squat position.

Duck Walk Relays

Put the kids in teams and have relay races where each kid first does duck walks with their hands on their hips. Then repeat with torpedo elbows. And then with the overhead positions. You can vary this exercise by doing a longer race with you have a course where, at every corner they turn, the kids have to change their hand position. Then you can give the winner a prize, such as the ability to choose the next game.

Musical Ducks and Grasshoppers

You know the drill. Same game, different characters. Change it up with whatever characters you want. You could make it so the winner of the last round chooses the character of the next round.

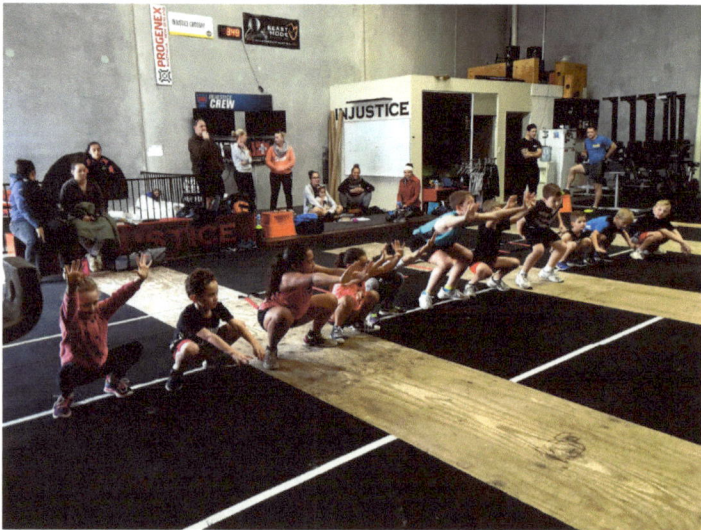

Finally, when the majority of the class knows this skill, you can test them with the following list:

Checklist to Pass "Duck Walks"

- Bottom close to heels

- Keep chest high

- Hands on hips

- Torpedo elbows

- Arms in overhead position

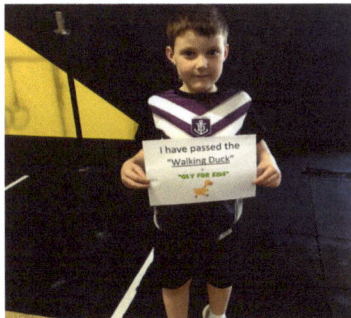

Recognition, Tracking, and Progress

At this point, I feel we should talk about progress. Throughout the programme, parents will come up to you and ask how their child is doing. How will you respond? Fortunately, with this programme measures and benchmarks are built into the system for you so that you can give the parents an accurate assessment. But to do that, you'll need to make sure you always have on hand a progress chart or something similar to record each child's progress.

With this book, I have included progress cards. You can print these out and give one to each child at the beginning of the programme. Write their name on it, and keep the cards together, either with you or at the gym. You could also create a wall poster chart or use a whiteboard to show the progress for all the kiddos to see at all times.

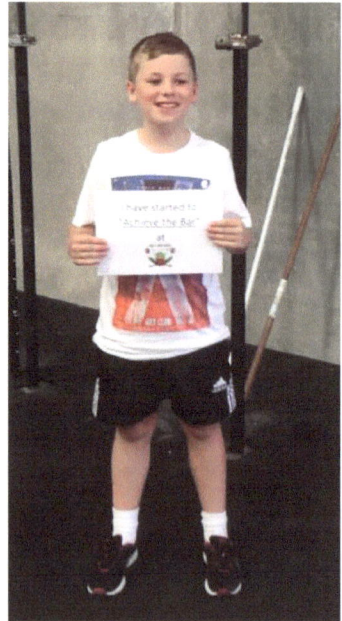

Here is an example of such a progress chart:

Achieve The Bar

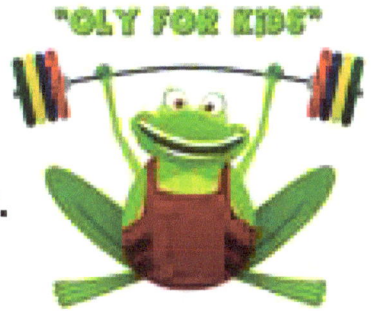
"OLY FOR KIDS"

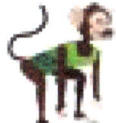
The Standing Monkey.

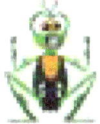
The Proud Grasshopper.

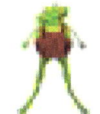
Jumping Frog.

Torpedo elbows.

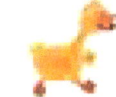
Duck walk.

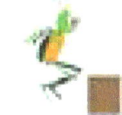
Box jumps.

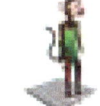
Ledge jumps.

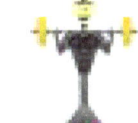
Larry the Lamppost.

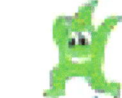
The Split Star Fish

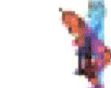
Robot Man

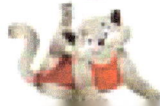
Stretchy Cat.

Oly4Kids

7. *Box Jumps*

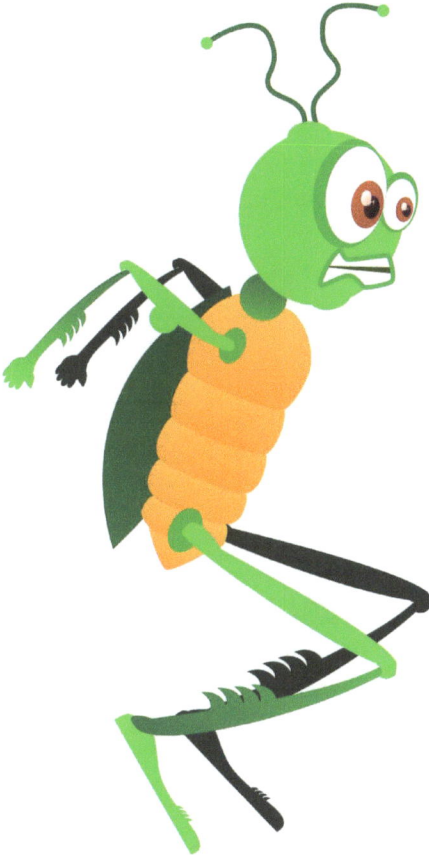

Although box jumps are not a specific part of the Oly lifts, they are key to the muscle development needed in this programme. The strength and explosiveness you learn and use in box jumps transfers over to the frog jump.

The important thing to remember with box jumps is to keep your core strong and stable. Bend the knees and then explode upwards while driving through the heels initially. As you leave the ground, push through the ball of the foot. It is best to use your arms to propel yourself then bring your feet up to meet the box as fast as you can. Then stand. Make it a tuck jump onto the box. An athlete will have a better clearance onto the box if the knees raise up to the chest as much as possible (this will help to prevent tripping onto the box or catching the toes on the edge).

This is a standard exercise and coaches will know how this goes. Just remember that with kids especially, it's important to start small and build up to bigger boxes and bigger jumps gradually.

Here are the learning outcome points you need:

- Feet about hip-width apart
- Bend knees and drive through the heels, but take off from the ball of the foot.
- Land on the box and straighten legs.

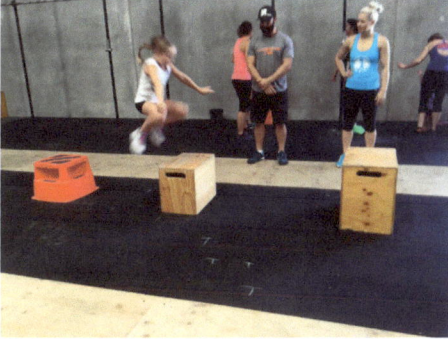

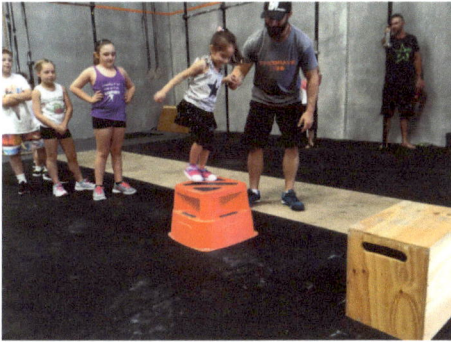

Here are ways to play with the kids to practice the box jumps.

Box Jump Ladder

Create two (or three, if class numbers make is necessary) box jump ladders of four or five boxes, starting from very low, like a bumper plate, up to very high. You want the biggest box to be a stretch; not every kid will do this. Also, I like to have coach assistants on either side of the box jump ladder so that if a child looks afraid and needs support, the assistants can be there to hold the child's hand. It is a very painful experience to graze your knee on the front of the box! If you have done this, you will agree. It would not be a good thing to give the child a fear of box jumps, as it is a very important exercise in developing explosive power.

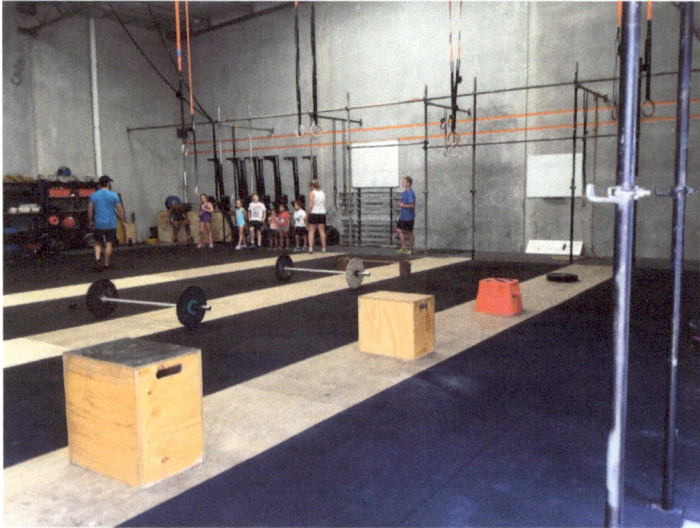

Box Jump Circuit Workout (or WOD)

Use box jump stations that are at a moderate height and suitable for the kids using them. So the little kids may just be jumping on a bumper plate. Bigger kids may be jumping on a medium height plate. The purpose of this exercise is to do the exercise over and over to develop the necessary skills and to feel familiar with it. An accident would only spoil things, so go lighter (lower box height) rather than harder (higher box height).

Finally, when the majority of the class knows this skill, you can test them with the following list:

Checklist to Pass "Box Jumps"

- Feet about hip width apart

- Use the jumping frog start position here (because the chest should start at an angle to get momentum to jump up)

- Bend knees with a flat back and high chest

- Drive through the heels, but push off from the ball of the foot

- Move feet to the box fast, with the focus on the knee drive to produce a faster movement

- Land and stand on straight knees

Oly4Kids

8. *Ledge Jumps*

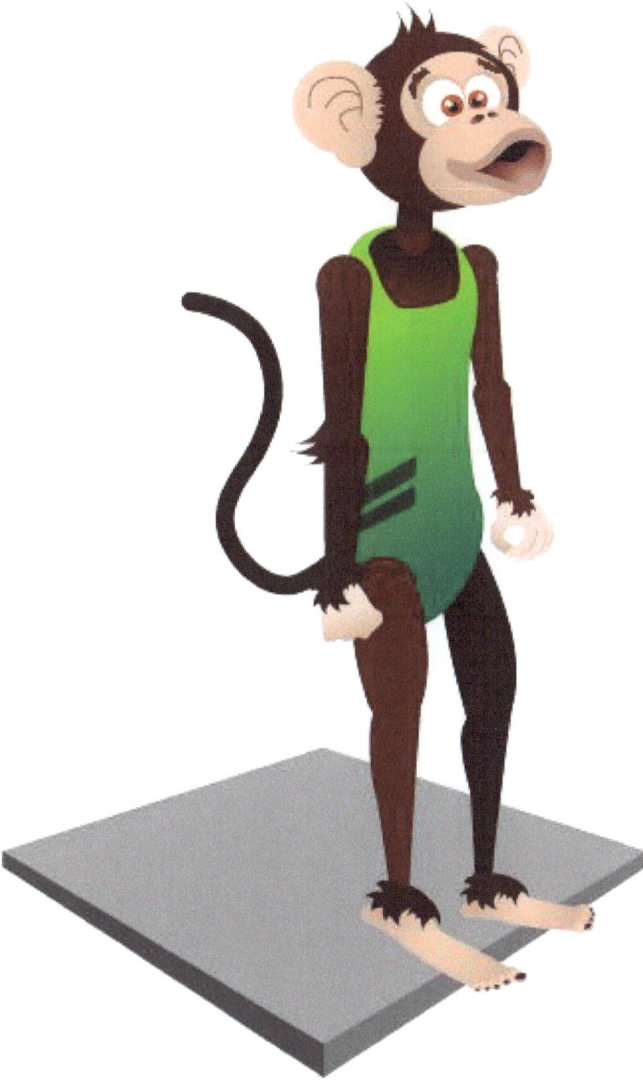

Teaching ledge jumps is important as it helps the kids to have the correct mind-body connection as they lift. When a lifter wants to drive the weight upwards, it is vital that they drive their force through the heels and not the balls of their feet. But it is difficult to get this idea across to athletes while teaching them the dip and drive position. But if you teach an athlete the dip while having him jump from a ledge which only supports the heels, he will no choice but to push through his heels. There is the added advantage that if they do not go straight up and straight down, they will not land as safely and solidly. That's why you put them on a ledge.

Now I should point out at this stage that the ledge cannot be any higher than about 10cm, the height of a competition platform. Obviously, we need to cater for kids not getting this right straight away, because believe me—adults don't, so why should kids? You want to make it safe so that when they miss the ledge on landing, it will only be a small step down to catch themselves. Any raised position can be used as a ledge. Even a larger bumper plate, like a 25kg plate, would suffice, although they do usually have a lip around the edge which would not make it easy to push from. So put some thought into what you can use as a ledge.

The learning outcome points are:

- Dip and drive on your heels.
- That's it!

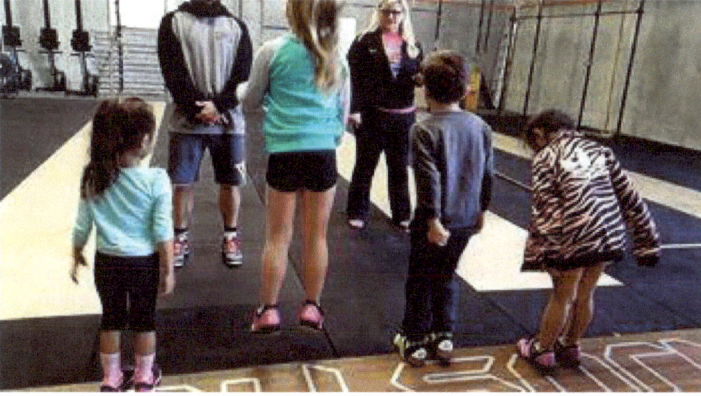

Ledge jumps are a small (but important) element of the Oly lifts, and so I have not come up with any games that practice this. I did find it was an exercise that took a while to wrap your head around, and we took lots of photos to demonstrate what the kids are doing, as opposed to what they thought they were doing. But this lesson is absolutely essential and one which should be taught to adult lifters, as well.

When you feel the majority of the class knows this skill, test them with the following list:

Checklist to Pass "Ledge Jumps"

- ■ Stand on heels on ledge with toes hanging over the edge

- ■ Bend knees with a flat back and high chest

- ■ Drive through the heels

- ■ Land back on your heels on the ledge

9. *Larry the Lamppost*

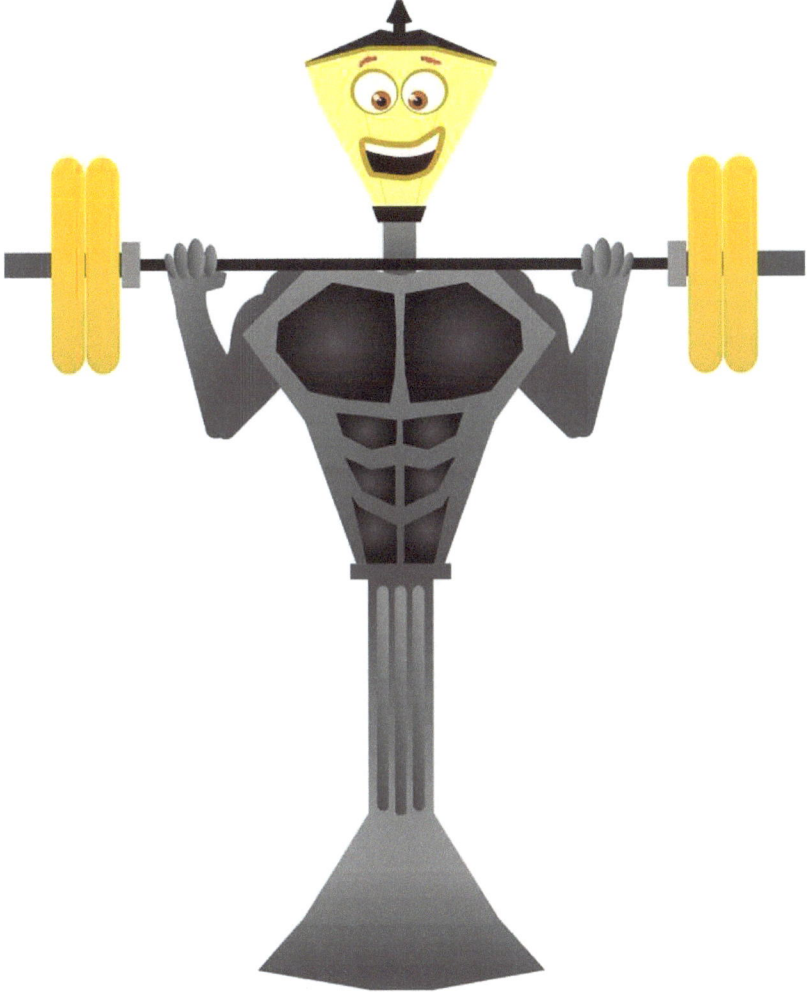

At first glance, it may seem like there is not much to consider when preparing for the jerk part of the clean & jerk lift. But there is! Preparation makes all the difference. Consider the act of holding a brick with a tennis ball on top of it and lifting the brick and ball upwards. Now contrast that with the act of holding onto a piece of rope (in place of the brick) with a tennis ball balancing on top and now trying to push the ball upwards. That rope will bend and change directions, making the ball travel in unplanned directions with little force. Similarly, when you lift, you need to prepare your back and torso so it is rigid and supportive like a brick and not like a rope. That is why I teach the kids to be a lamppost.

Let's chunk it down. The students need to stand in the rack position: feet shoulder width apart, hands outside the shoulders, and chest up. Start from the ground. The feet must be apart, turned out a bit, and the weight solidly back on the heels—not on the balls of the feet, as this will create forward movement when they dip. The knees must start locked. The bottom should be tight and clenched hard. I always ask them to pretend they are holding a coin between their cheeks. (This always creates a lot of laughter). The abdominal muscles must be tight to give good core stability. Fill the lungs with air and hold the chest high.

So now we have created the post. Whether a lamppost is made of wood or metal, it will not bend or sway, so it gives the right notion for the child to have a good, tight starting position.
The arms should ideally be out with the elbows pointing down (although still slightly forward) before the jerk, but not everyone can do this. The most important thing is that the chest is high and the shoulders are back and under the bar. That way the lifter is able to drive the bar upwards. Elbows down creates the best position for the arms to go in a straight

line upwards. It is important to note here that the arms are not pressing the weight of the bar upwards—the legs are doing this. The arms are merely limbs to guide and then catch the bar at the full upward extension position. This is very important from a technical point of view because any press out in the jerk movement in a competition will result in a no lift.

Next, you will want to teach the dip. This needs to be performed with the weight remaining on the heels, chest high and the torso tight. Both the glutes and the abs should stay clenched as you dip to keep that integrity in your torso. (Tell the kiddos that they need to be able to dip without dropping that coin between the cheeks.) The dip should be short, controlled, and precise. Some lifters have the tendency to dip fast, but it is the drive that must be fast. Other lifters have the tendency to dip long, but it is the drive that must be long. Don't get those two mixed up. The lifter needs to differentiate the speed and intensity between the dip and the drive.

The last part of the Lamppost is the drive. Once you have dipped straight and tight, you need to then change directions and drive upwards. Once again the force must be going through the heel, not the ball of the foot. This is why we covered the ledge jumps before coming to the Lamppost. The principle of having all your weight on the heels and driving through the heels cannot be understated! It changes efficiency, effectiveness, and direction. Everything we talk about in Oly is about the lines and movement path that have the greatest efficiency. While the dip is short and controlled, the drive has to be fast and long, to gain the maximum momentum out of it.

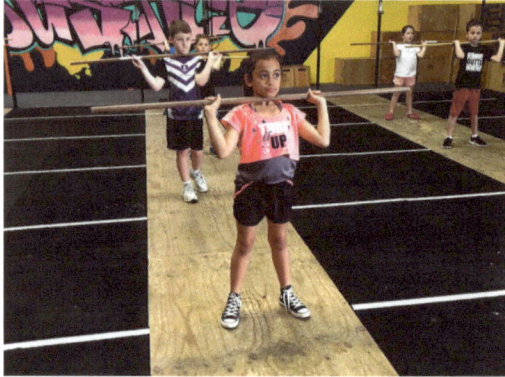

Here are the learning outcome points you need to cover:

- Feet shoulder width apart
- Keep chest high
- Hands outside shoulders
- Elbows down and shoulders under the bar
- Dip on the heels with tight core (bottom, abs, and chest)
- Drive off the heels, and drive fast and long

Here are ways to play with the kids to practice the Lamppost.

Musical Lampposts and Grasshoppers

You know the drill. Same game, different characters. Change it up with whatever characters you want. You could make it the winner of the last round chooses the character of the next round and the winner.

Ladder of Standing Monkey, Jumping Frog, Proud Grasshopper, and Lamppost

Use stations that are marked with a line, spaced out so they fill the length of the space you have to work in. If possible, have something up high at the last station for the kids to reach up and touch after they had done their dip and drive from the lamppost. This could be an object like a bell or even an adult's hand to high five. What this game does is put a clean and jerk together (almost).

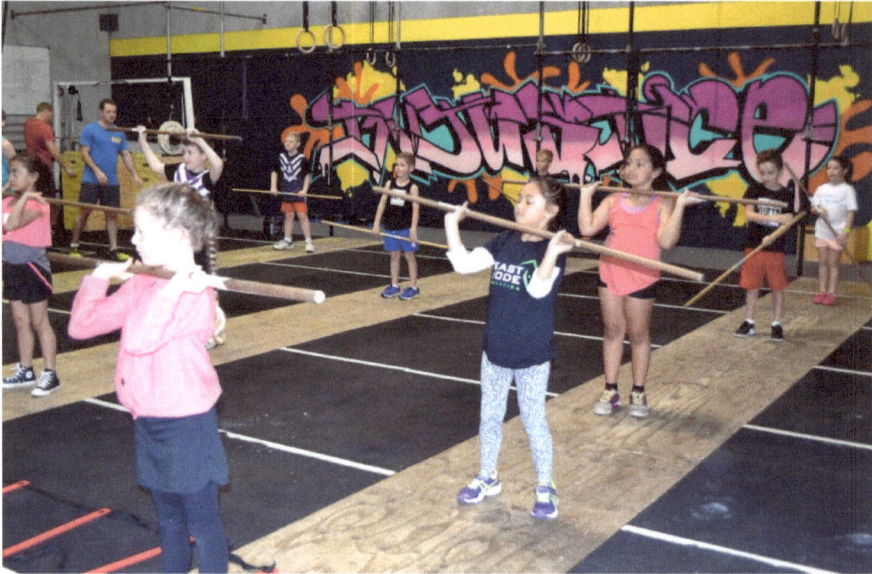

Finally, when the majority of the class knows this skill, test them with the following list:

Checklist to Pass "The Lamppost"

- Feet shoulder width apart

- Keep chest high

- Hands outside shoulders

- Elbows down and shoulders under the bar

- Dip on the heels with tight core (bottom, abs, and chest)

- Drive off the heels, and drive fast and long

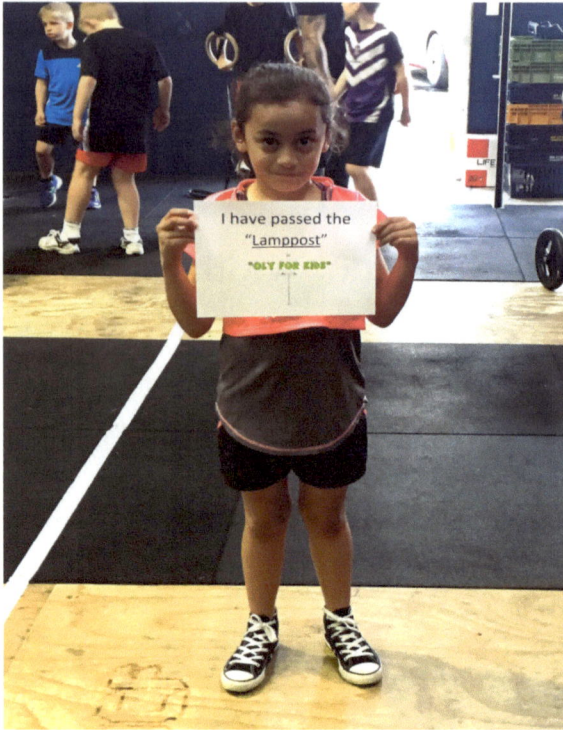

10. The Split Starfish

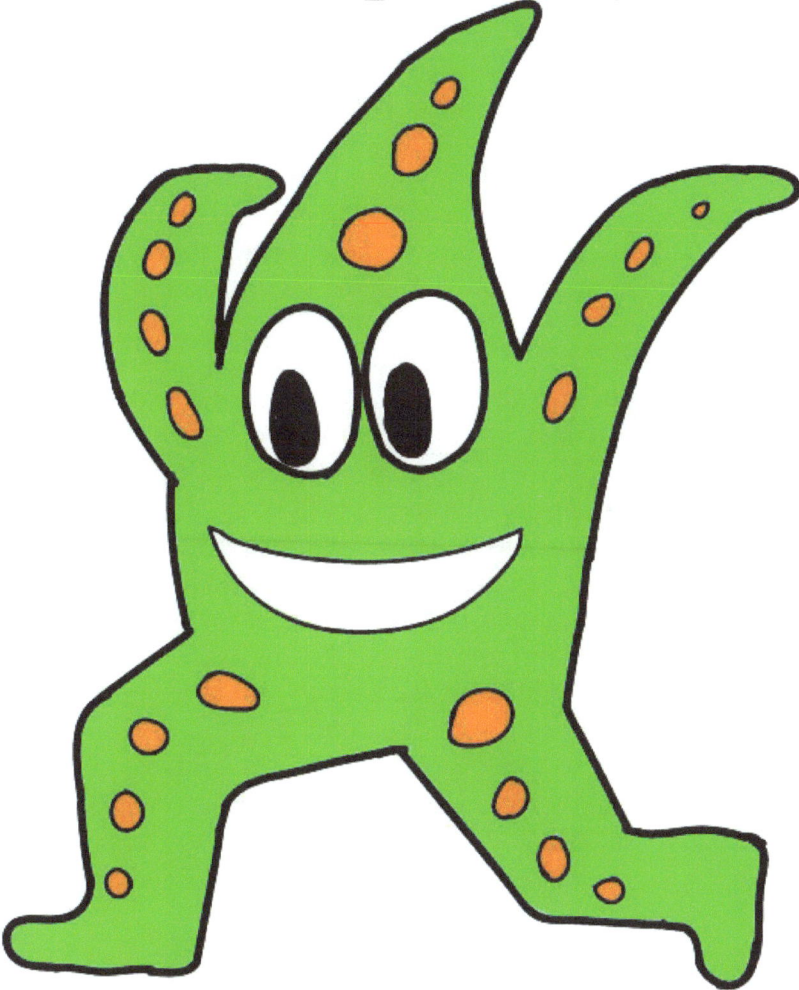

In this section, we will learn how to master the jerk split position. After you have done the Lamppost dip and drive, now you need to know exactly how you want to position your body for the jerk split, or as we call it, the Split Starfish. The reason I use this name is because there are two things you need to keep in mind for this movement: how you position your legs and arms.

Teach this position with the child standing on a drawn square on the ground. Chalk is handy for this exercise. The start position for the split with your two feet shoulder-width apart and slightly turned out. The feet should be right in the middle of the box, as shown below. Then, after you dip and drive from that position, your feet should jump out equidistant forward and backwards. Emphasize this point as many new lifters move the back foot further than the front foot. If the lifter goes too far back, she could move the bar too much, destabilizing it overhead. Also, make sure the lifter keeps her feet tipped slightly outward, with her back knee slightly bent and the back heel raised to allow for compensation movements. Her hips should be right under the bar.

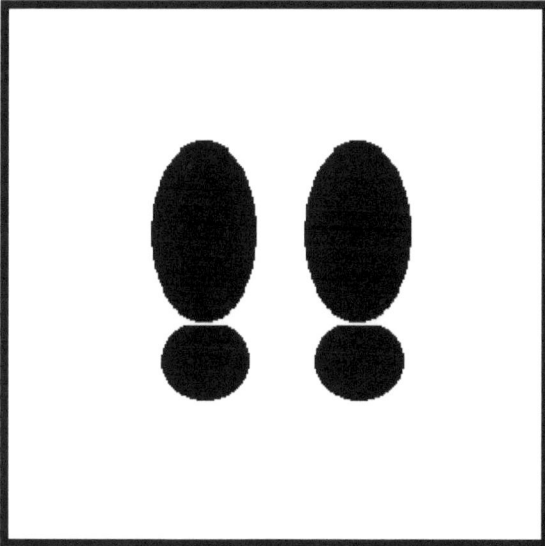

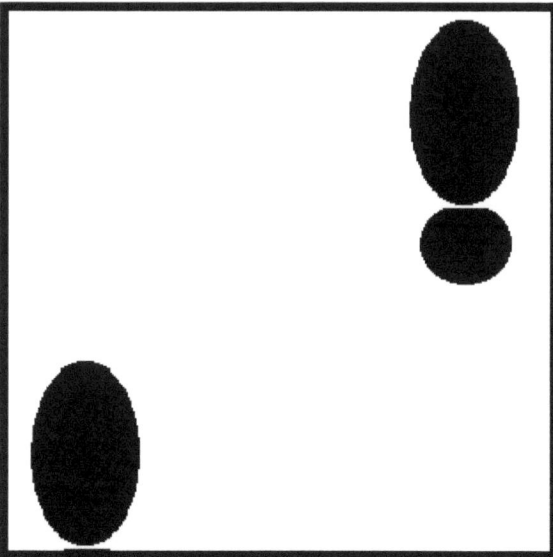

The last part of this is the recovery from the jerk split. When bringing the feet back together, the best practice is to pull the front foot back in, halfway to the start position. Then bring the back foot in, and lastly move the front foot again so you are in the start position. There is a very good reason for this. When you pull the front foot back in incrementally, the bar stays in the same position overhead. But if you were to bring the back foot in first, this tends to give the bar forward momentum, causing you to lose the jerk forward. Also, it is much easier to move the back foot first, so the lifter may take a bigger step than if she used her front foot.

Be sure to cover the following learning outcome points, which are:

- Feet shoulder width apart, in the middle of the square
- Dip and drive on your heels
- Split the feet, equidistant forward and backwards, to fill the box
- Hands go from the shoulders to a star position
- Back leg bent and heel raised
- Recovery front foot first

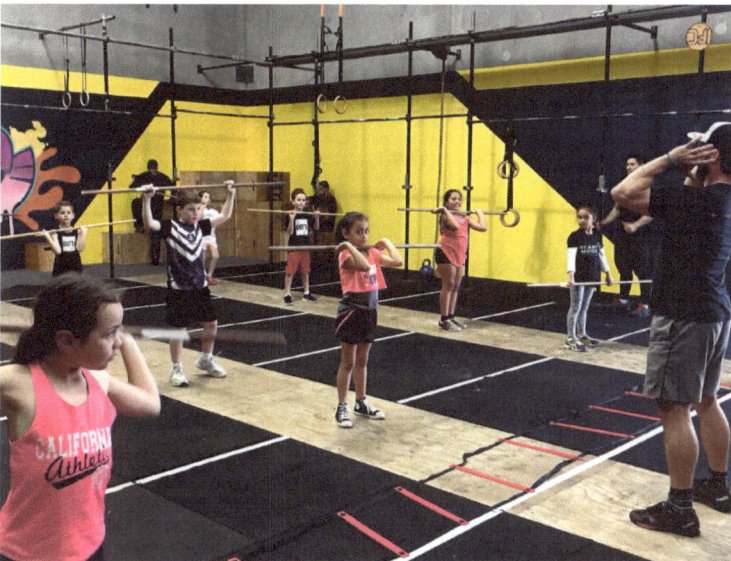

Here are ways to play with the kids to practice the Split Starfish.

Musical Split Starfish

You know the drill. Same game, different characters. The only difference with this one is that is better to have the kids jumping on two feet so when the music stops, they are in the right position to split. Jumping within their square would be best, but you could also make it that they have to find a square, jump on two feet, and then split star.

Ladder of Standing Monkey, Jumping Frog, Proud Grasshopper, Lamppost and Split Star

Use stations that are marked with a line, spaced out so they fill the length of the space you have to work in. If possible, have something up high at the last station for the kids to reach up and touch after they had done their dip and drive from the Lamppost. You can use either an object like a bell or just an adult's hand to high five. What this game does is put a clean and jerk together, complete with the jerk this time.

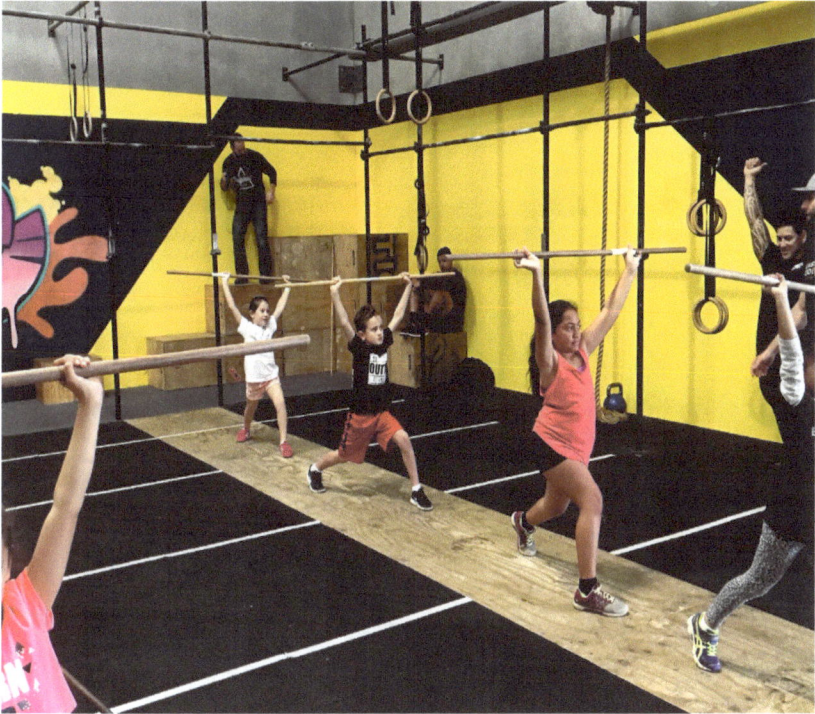

When the majority of the class knows this skill, you can test them with the following list:

Checklist to Pass "The Split Starfish"

- Feet shoulder width apart, in the middle of the square

- Dip and drive on your heels

- Split the feet, equidistant forward and backwards, to fill the box

- Hands go from the shoulders to a star position

- Back leg bent and heel raised

- Recovery front foot first

11. Robot Man

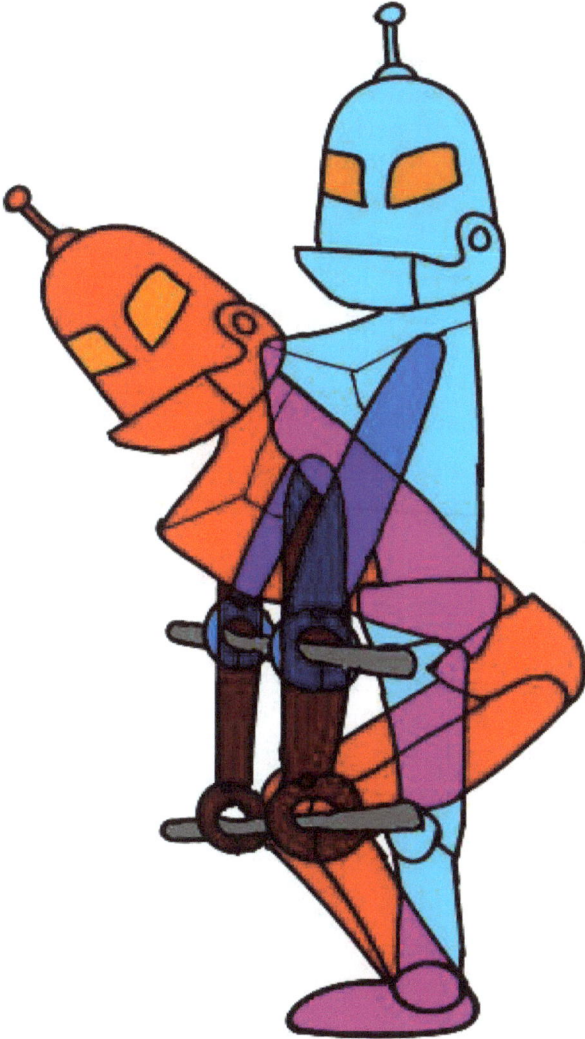

Now we can put all of our learned positions and movements together!

Using the Robot Man character, we will assimilate all the movements we've learned with precision. Going through the lifting movements properly is all about locking the core and being very mindful about where all your body parts go. This is something that was taught to me late in my weightlifting education and it has brought everything else together for me, helping me to get a good feel for the correct Oly positions and understand the science behind it. Once you have learned all the correct Oly positions and movements and then proceed to use them in the Oly lifts, you will feel surprisingly a bit like a robot. Kids get that feeling—they like it, understand it, and will embrace the precision and the discipline of a robot to practise their lifts.

Since this part is a culmination of all the other parts of this programme, I will talk about the movements step by step. You will notice that we have covered all areas of the clean and jerk except how to get to the Standing Monkey. We talked at length about being in the position, but now we will start the moves from standing straight up.

Let's put this all together.

- Start in a standing position with feet shoulder-width apart, feet slightly turned out.
- With a straight back, push your bottom backwards, whilst keeping your chest proud.
- When you get to the position whereby your bottom is backwards as far as your chest is forwards, then it is time to stop pushing the bottom backwards, and now bend the knees to continue lowering the body until your

arms (whilst hanging downward) reach the bar.

- At this point, you should be in the Standing Monkey (flat back, chest over bar, neck in line with the spine whilst looking slightly forward).
- Once you grab the bar, you then do all that in reverse—straighten the knees, and bring the bottom back in to lock the hips.
- You then follow this through with a shrug of the shoulders to do the Jumping Frog.
- Once the bar passes your torso in this upward movement, engage your Torpedo Elbows and Proud Grasshopper.
- Keeping Torpedo Elbows forward, stand into the Lamppost. The elbows go down only when you are ready to dip and drive.
- Next, dip and drive on your heels like the ledge jump and land in the Split Starfish, with the bar overhead.
- Lastly, recovery—front foot first.

Checklist to Pass "Robot Man"

■ Start in a standing position with feet shoulder-width apart, feet slightly turned out.

■ With a straight back and proud chest, push your bottom backwards.

■ When you get to the position whereby your bottom is backwards as far as your chest is forwards, then it is time to stop pushing the bottom backwards, and now bend the knees to continue lowering the body until your arms (whilst hanging downward) reach the bar.

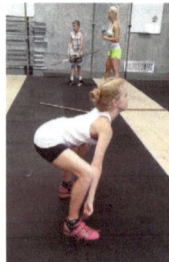

The Wrap Up

Let us summarize what we have learnt over this ten-week period.

We have covered the eleven stages of learning, each of which has taught us a particular skill, movement, or technique which will eventually become part of the two Olympic weightlifting movements—the snatch and the clean & jerk. Each one of these stages plays a particular role in the big picture, although on their own it may not seem like it.

The main principles of the "Oly 4 Kids" programme are technique, consistency, repetition, muscle memory, mobility, core strength and stability, long-term good habits, and most of all—a lot of fun! My intention was to make weightlifting fun and interesting for kids. The programme is full of recognition and reinforcement. It is always important to take the time to make every child know that they're special, for whatever they are good at. Kids love to have their photo taken, so I have worked that into each level, so they can feel they have accomplished something.

Once a child has completed all the levels satisfactorily, they are ready to go on to Part 2 - "Controlling the Bar". In this part, the students will connect the positions and movements that they learnt through the "Oly 4 Kids" characters into exercises which form part of a weightlifting athlete's workout. Although we still do not lift any significant weight, as we are still learning, young bodies need to practise the proper technique to apply additional weight to the bar in the future.

I hope you will see how advantageous this programme is to the development of children, to the benefit of their growing physique and their sporting abilities. It promotes core strength, muscle control, concentration, and muscle stamina. It also is the building blocks to having explosive, fast power. Strength in a controlled environment is what we are working towards.

If you are interested in following "Oly 4 Kids", they can be found at www.Oly4Kids.com.au and on Facebook at Oly 4 Kids. I plan to put up resources for members, such as the "I have achieved …" placards, the programme tracking cards, and other great stuff.

See you online, Oly friends!

www.ingramcontent.com/pod-product-compliance
Lightning Source LLC
Chambersburg PA
CBHW040929030426
42334CB00002B/18